Testosterone: A Man's Guide

Practical Tips for Boosting Sexual, Physical, and Mental Vitality

Nelson Vergel, BsChE, MBA
Co-Author of "Built To Survive"

Disclaimer

The information contained in this publication is for educational purposes only, and is in no way a substitute for the advice of a qualified health care provider. Appropriate medical therapy and the use of pharmaceutical compounds like testosterone should be tailored for the individual, as no two individuals are alike. The author does not recommend self-medicating with any compound, as you should consult with a qualified medical doctor who can determine your individual situation. Any use of the information presented in this publication for personal medical therapy is done strictly at your own risk and no responsibility is implied or intended on the part of the author, contributors, or the publisher.

Cover Design: Rob Tomlin, Houston, Texas
Vergel, Nelson, 1959
Testosterone: A Man's Guide
First edition
ISBN: 978-0966223125
Medicine, Health, Nutrition, Chemistry, Endocrinology
Library of Congress Control Number: 2010933334

Milestones Publishing
P.O. Box 667223
Houston, TX 77266

For updates, visit **TestosteroneWisdom.com**

I would like to thank my partner Timothy Baker, MD for his support and the many hours he spent to help me editing this book. I would also like to thank my friends Bonnie Goldman for editing and giving me pointers about what an interesting book should look like and Rob Tomlin for his great cover design work. And last but not least, thanks to all the people in the past 20 years who I have met in my lectures and online forums that have shared their health tips so that others could walk on an easier road in their search for health. I hope I have become a vessel for all that communal wisdom to be offered to the world.

ABOUT THE AUTHOR

Nelson Vergel is the co-author of the book "Built to Survive: A Comprehensive Guide on the Medical Use of Anabolic Therapies, Nutrition and Exercise for HIV+ Women and Men" and the founder of the Body Positive Wellness Clinic in Houston. He holds a bachelor's degree in chemical engineering from McGill University and an MBA from the University of Houston. A tireless patient advocate for over 20 years, his writing is accessible and jam-packed full of practical information. He weaves the latest research data with first-hand experience and useful tips—the result of years of trial and error experience. He strives to help his readers live healthier lives without having to "reinvent the wheel" in their search for solutions.

Nelson discovered the benefits of testosterone replacement therapy in 1993 after doing his own research to reverse his death threatening spiral with fatigue and wasting syndrome. Testosterone allowed him to regain his health as he built lean body mass and regained his energy. This in turn bought him time to survive HIV until effective therapies were introduced in 1996. Convinced that testosterone saved him from dying of wasting, he embarked on a lecture crusade that has helped thousands of people live healthier lives through the medical use of hormones, exercise, nutrition, supplementation, and other wellness-related therapies. He also was honored to join respectable research team on the subject of metabolism and illness.

After spending four years as an active member of metabolic disorders research committee at AIDS Clinical Trials Group of the U. S. National Institutes of Health, he became a leading treatment advocate and has been featured in numerous publications for his expertise and perspective. He has lectured at over 60 scientific conferences and to over 500 physician and patient groups, is an expert advisor at TheBody.com, and actively manages the largest online health support group for those living with HIV (pozhealth at yahoogroups.com). Because of his dedicated efforts to help others, the Mayor of the City of Houston, Lee Brown, proclaimed September 13, 2001as "Nelson Vergel Day."

In this book, Nelson wants to share his 27 years of survival and health wisdom with men around the world, regardless of their health status. The time has come for all men regardless of health status to learn from what he and others have gathered in their years of health struggles. It is his hope that no man has to suffer needlessly from a condition that is easily treatable if monitored by a properly trained physician.

ABBREVIATIONS

Androgen Deficiency in the Aging Male	ADAM
benign prostatic hyperplasia	BPH
dehydroepiandrosterone	DHEA
dihydrotestosterone	DHT
digital rectal examination	DRE
Drug Enforcement Agency	DEA
estrogen receptor	ER
follicle-stimulating hormone	FSH
Food and Drug Administration	FDA
free testosterone	FT
gonadotropin-releasing hormone	GnRH
health management organization	HMO
high-density lipoprotein	HDL
highly active antiretroviral therapy	HAART
human chorionic gonadotropin	HCG
human growth hormone	HGH
hypothalamic-pituitary-gonadal axis	HPGA
hypothalamic-pituitary-testicular axis	HPTA
low density lipoprotein	LDL
luteinizing hormone	LH
nitric oxide	NO
over-the-counter	OTC
Physician's Desk Reference	PDR
prostatic specific antigen	PSA
selective androgen receptor modulators	SARMs
sex hormone binding globulin	SHBG
stopping anabolic steroids	SAS
testosterone replacement therapy	TR

TABLE OF CONTENTS

LIST OF FIGURES

Introduction

My relationship with hormonal replacement has been a long and fruitful one. I was diagnosed with low testosterone in 1993 at the age of 34 after I had been living with HIV for 11 years. I had lost 14 pounds unintentionally, felt tired and depressed, and had no sex drive at all. I was convinced that it was the beginning of the end for me. Many of my friends with HIV began looking like skeletons due to wasting syndrome, a severe unintentional loss of body weight. And then many died. I was starting to buy into the myth that feeling tired and ending up in bones were normal if one is HIV+.

Luckily in Los Angeles I met HIV+ guys in support groups who were already using testosterone in an underground manner. They boasted about how great they felt and looked. At the time I was terrified to consider the hormone since I had heard that it caused liver and prostate cancer, destroyed one's immune system, and that it would supposedly induce horrible "steroid rage." I was finally convinced to take an educated risk when my fear of dying of wasting became stronger than my fears of testosterone.

I was able to get some testosterone cypionate and had a friend help me inject 200 mg of it in my upper buttock. After two injections (a week apart), I started to improve: My mind was less foggy, my sex drive was returning, my depression lessened, and my weight loss stabilized. I felt like I was alive again and regained my appetite not only for food, but for life itself. What I thought were symptoms of immune dysfunction were symptoms of having low testosterone. I began to feel like a healthy 34-year old should. With the help of exercise and proper nutrition, I was able to gain 35 pounds of lean body mass, even with uncontrolled HIV virus in my blood. I had hope again.

My amazing transformation inspired me to read all I could about testosterone and androgens in medical journals. This started a journey that has taken me through 16 years of self-education on the subject. In 1999 I co-wrote a book called "Built To Survive: A Comprehensive Guide to the Medical Use of Anabolic Hormones" with Michael Mooney on the medical uses of androgens, exercise, and nutrition to reverse HIV-related wasting and to improve quality of life. After that book was launched, I received many emails from healthy HIV-negative men with questions about testosterone. I realized that the information we gathered in HIV was invaluable also for men without the virus. So I decided to write this book for *all* men who need help, regardless of their health status.

Since its discovery in the early 20th century, the world has learned a lot about testosterone. Unfortunately testosterone is probably also one of the most misunderstood hormones in medicine. Stigma, denial and misconceptions have been barriers for most men to consider its use—even in the presence of all the debilitating symptoms of testosterone deficiency (hypogonadism). These fears have been fueled by a media that equates testosterone supplementation with aggression and with the athletes who abuse it, as well as by physicians who have a poor understanding of testosterone replacement therapy (TRT).

Results from one of the largest studies ever done on testosterone deficiency, the Hypogonadism in Males (HIM) study published in 2006, estimated the overall prevalence of hypogonadism in the United States at approximately 39 percent in men aged 45 years or older. Recent estimates show that 13 million men in the United States may experience testosterone deficiency, although fewer than 10 percent receive treatment for the condition. So why are so many men receiving treatment for hypogonadism?

Consider that men are known *not* to proactively visit doctors. And consider that the two main symptoms of testosterone deficiency, depression and sexual dysfunction, are topics that most men feel uncomfortable discussing even with their physicians. So even if he is feeling bad enough to finally make it to the doctor, a man is probably more willing to take a physical gut punch than the metaphorical one by admitting out loud that he has problems with his sexual performance or his mood.

Many men suffer needlessly with these problems that dramatically affect their quality of life and how they relate to others. Depression and sexual dysfunction both have been linked to cardiovascular risks factors that affect not only the length of life but more importantly, its quality. Growing older while remaining healthy and independent is surely everyone's wish. This book will provide one of the pieces of the puzzle on how to attain this goal.

Since my last book, several studies have demonstrated that testosterone is an important and relatively safe hormone for those with testosterone deficiency who are monitored by a trained physician. New products like testosterone gels have entered the market and have helped raise testosterone literacy among physicians. But demonization of this hormone and its cousin molecules, anabolic steroids, has not gone away, mostly due to unfounded fears based on lack of information. Regrettably, the media and the U.S. Congress have focused on the use of testosterone by athletes who utilize these compounds at high doses *without* consulting trained physicians. This media hysteria may also add to the fears about testosterone's side effects present in the minds of potential patients living with hypogonadism who are suffering needlessly and quietly.

Besides researching data on different options, I have purposely tried most of the products that I discuss in this book to provide practical tips on each. I have also been lucky to learn from experiences of many people using these products via my online listserve and lectures in the past 16 years. It is my hope that this book will save readers time and trouble by preventing costly mistakes, wasted time and needless suffering. I tried to write it in accessible language. My suggestions are not intended to be medical advice and I strongly urge every reader to seek the opinion of a qualified and trained physician before engaging in any of the health solutions reviewed in this book.

I have also included valuable information on patient assistance programs and how to find physicians trained in testosterone replacement therapy to save valuable time and money for men searching for solutions to their hypogonadism.

Even though this book focuses on men, you will notice that I included some information about testosterone in women. As of 2010, there is no Food Drug Administration (FDA) approved testosterone product for women, although many doctors have been prescribing small doses in specially compounded creams for lack of libido in females. There are even some products in studies and close to potential approval for women.

Please do not hesitate to email me via my web site TestosteroneWisdom. com, a site created to provide updates on new information as it becomes available. Also, please let me know what you think by posting your review on amazon.com.

Wishing you the best health and prosperity,

Nelson Vergel

Testosterone 101

History of Testosterone

Since man has been walking upright and letting it all hang out, there has been fascination and misinformation about those things that make him male. There were the early beliefs that the eating of penis or testicles from animals was a way to improve virility (still apparently goes on in some parts of the world, given the market for rhino and seal penis). This awareness of the role of the testicles in sexual functioning laid the groundwork for men of science to get involved, sometimes in unusual ways.

In 1889 Charles Edouard Brown-Sequard created a liquid extract made from dog testicles, reporting that it increased his strength. In 1918 Leo L. Stanley transplanted testicles that had been removed from recently executed San Quentin State prisoners into their still living fellow inmates, some of whom claimed improved sexual potency. In the 1920s the French-Russian surgeon Serge Voronoff, made a fortune grafting testicular monkey tissue onto the testicles of aging men.

It wasn't until 1935 that Karoly G. David and Ernst Laqueur isolated crystalline testosterone from testicles. Shortly afterwards, two different groups led by Adolf Butenandt and Leopold Ruzicka developed synthetic methods of preparing testosterone. Butenandt and Ruzicka shared the 1939 Nobel Prize in chemistry for this achievement., going to show you that not only will we men give our junk a name but given the chance, also a really, really big prize.

These early formulations of testosterone were quickly broken down in the body. It wasn't until the development of testosterone esters (i.e., a type of chemical compound designed to slow down the breakdown of testosterone in the body) in the 1950s and 1960s that more scientific studies could eventually be done that showed the improved muscle mass and strength, libido, energy, bone density, and overall well-being associated with testosterone replacement therapy.

What Is Testosterone and How Does It Work?

Testosterone is the hormone responsible for normal growth and development and maintenance of male sex characteristics. It also affects lean body mass, mood and sexual function in both males and females. It is the primary androgenic (responsible for masculine characteristics) and anabolic (muscle building) hormone.

Testosterone is produced by the testicles in males and by the ovaries in females, with small amounts also produced by the adrenal glands in both genders. Its production and secretion are regulated by other hormones in a hormonal cascade.

Figure 1. Hormonal cascade that regulates testosterone production in males

As shown in Figure 1, the hormonal and reproductive function of the testicles (gonads) is regulated through interactions among the hypothalamus, the pituitary gland, and the gonads (commonly known as the hypothalamic-pituitary-gonadal axis [HPGA]). The three glands communicate through a cascade of hormones and a self-regulating feedback loop that controls the generation of each hormone. Release of gonadotropin-releasing hormone (GnRH) from the hypothalamus regulates secretion of other hormones (gonadotropins) that influence the testicles by way of the pituitary. GnRH controls the secretion of luteinizing hormone (LH) and follicle-stimulating hormone (FSH) by the anterior pituitary. Luteinizing hormone regulates the production and secretion of testosterone through the Leydig cells of the testes, while FSH stimulates the production of sperm.

When someone is found to have low testosterone blood levels this is known as "hypogonadism" There are several types of hypogonadism:

- Primary hypogonadism is a hypergonadotropic condition (higher than normal levels of LH and FSH). This occurs when the testicles fail to produce sufficient levels of testosterone to suppress production of LH and FSH. As a result, LH and FSH levels are elevated while testosterone levels are decreased. The pituitary glands tried to increase testosterone at no avail even after increasing LH and FSH.

- **Secondary hypogonadism** results from hypothalamic or pituitary dysfunction. It is characterized by disruption of central components of the HPGA resulting in decreased levels of GnRH, LH, or FSH. In this type of hypogonadism, low levels of LH do not allow for the proper stimulation of the production of testosterone by the testes.

- **Mixed hypogonadism** results from a combination of primary and secondary causes. The most common cause of mixed hypogonadism is late-onset hypogonadism, which occurs with aging. This is associated with osteoporosis, decreased lean body mass, reduced cognition, fatigue and impairment of libido and erectile function. Other causes of mixed hypogonadism include alcoholism, diseases (such as uremia, liver failure, AIDS, and sickle cell disease), street drugs/alcohol, and medications like corticosteroid steroids used for inflammatory conditions. It should be noted that high levels of cortisol (hypercortisolism), resulting from either the use of anti-inflammatory steroids or physical causes, could lead to hypogonadism.

As shown in Figure 2, testosterone in the body can convert into other hormones and metabolites. The process in which testosterone is converted into estrogen (a female hormone) by the aromatase enzyme is known as "aromatization". Males with high body fat, aging males, males taking certain medications, Males with sex chromosome genetic conditions such as Klinefelters Syndrome or males with a genetic disposition to having higher than normal amounts of aromatase may experience higher conversion of testosterone into estrogen. Estrogen blood levels are usually measured by detecting estradiol, the main estrogen in humans.

Testosterone Metabolites and Their Functions

Figure 2: Testosterone Metabolites

Estrogen is a very important hormone for men at the right concentration. It plays an important role in bone, hair, skin, and brain health as well as other functions in men. Large amounts of estrogen can cause mood swings, enlarged breasts (gynecomastia), fat gain, and water retention.

Another metabolite of testosterone is dihydrotestosterone (DHT). DHT has a positive effect on sexual desire but increases the production of excess skin oil, which can cause acne, hair loss, and prostatic inflammation.

So, it is important to monitor and determine the proper dosage of testosterone so that estradiol and DHT are kept within reference ranges needed for healthy body function as well as to prevent unwanted side effects of TRT.

As shown in Figure 3, about 2 percent of the testosterone in the body is active. This "free testosterone" is not attached to binding proteins that would prevent it from interacting with its receptor.

About 40 percent of the body's testosterone is attached to albumin. This is a protein that can release the hormone as the need for it arises in the body. Free testosterone and testosterone attached to albumin are referred to as "bioavailable testosterone".

In a healthy young male, about 60 percent of his testosterone is attached to sex hormone binding globulin (SHBG). Hormones bound to SHBG can't be used by the body and lose their anabolic effect. As males grow older or if illness is present, SHBG sweeps up more and more testosterone, lowering free testosterone and its benefits.

Total testosterone is the sum of bioavailable testosterone and testosterone bound to SHBG. Measuring just the total testosterone in the blood may not provide the whole picture and let you know how much "active" or usable testosterone you have.

Figure 3. Testosterone fractions in the blood

The normal levels of combined bound and free testosterones in male bodies can range anywhere from 300 to 1,100 ng/dL (nanograms per deciliter). Levels will vary with age and individual factors. It is useful to also measure the level of free testosterone as this may be more indicative of how hormone therapy is progressing. Levels of free testosterone can range between 0.3 and 5 percent of the total testosterone count, with about 2 percent considered an optimal level.

Higher than normal testosterone (i.e., above 1,100 ng/dL of total testosterone) can cause hair loss, acne, mood swings, mania in those with bipolar disorder, water retention, breast enlargement in men, increased aggression and hypersexual behavior, potential prostatic inflammation in older men, increases in the bad cholesterol (low density lipoprotein [LDL]), and decreases in the good cholesterol (high density lipoprotein [HDL]). Like everything in life, balance is key. Too much of a good thing can be detrimental.

Proper monitoring by an experienced physician is extremely important to ensure optimal levels of testosterone, to maximize benefits and to minimize side effects.

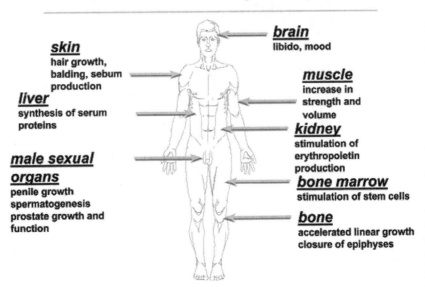

Figure 4 Target organs for beneficial and negative effects of testosterone (Courtesy of Dr. Donald Abrams)

What Are the Symptoms of Low Testosterone (Deficiency)?

As mentioned previously, hypogonadism is the medical term for the condition in males that is caused when the body is not producing sufficient amounts of testosterone. What most people don't realize is that in addition to sexual desire, testosterone also affects lean body mass, strength, bone density, mental focus, mood, fat loss, and other important factors in both males **and** females (Figure 4).

Common complaints for men with hypogonadism include: lower sexual desire (libido), erectile dysfunction (softer erections or lack of erections), depression, low energy and appetite, changes in body composition (lower lean body mass and higher abdominal fat), lower strength, reductions in body and facial hair, less mental focus and decreased height and osteoporosis (decrease in bone density).

As Table 1 shows, normalizing testosterone in people who have lower than normal levels has dramatic benefits, among which are increased sexual desire, lean body mass, bone density, strength, mood, motivation, mental focus, and stamina. However, these benefits can be erased if proper monitoring, dose adjustment, and appropriate choice of testosterone replacement option are not accomplished.

Table 1. Benefits of Normalizing Testosterone

Restored sexual desire
Improved erectile function
Improved mood/ sense of wellbeing
Increased lean body mass, strength and stamina
Improved bone density
Decreased fat mass

Determining If You Have Testosterone Deficiency

In addition to blood tests and physical examination, a brief screening instrument has also been developed by researchers at St. Louis University to aid in the diagnosis of hypogonadism. Known as the Androgen Deficiency in the Aging Male (ADAM) questionnaire:

1. Do you have a decrease in sex drive?
2. Do you lack energy?
3. Have you experienced a decrease in strength and/or endurance?
4. Do you feel shorter? Have you lost height? (Lower bone density can decrease height.)
5. Have you noticed a decreased enjoyment of life?
6. Are you sad and/or grumpy?
7. Are your erections less strong or gone?
8. Has it been more difficult to maintain your erection throughout sexual intercourse?
9. Are you falling asleep after dinner?
10. Has your work performance deteriorated recently?

Other questions that are usually not asked by doctors, but which I've found to be important are the following:

- Are you relating well with people around you?
- Are you being loving to your lover or life partner?
- Are you able to pay attention when someone talks to you?

In my life low testosterone caused problems that went far beyond sex and my body. It affected the way that I related to people and my ability to handle stress at work and in life.

Note that several of the above-mentioned problems can be caused by many other issues unrelated to low testosterone. Depression, anxiety, stress, medications and/or sleep disorders can cause nine of those 10 symptoms (decrease in height would be the only item unrelated to anything but bone loss or back surgery). This questionnaire is not a perfect predictor of low testosterone and should not replace tests for testosterone blood levels.

The benefit of this questionnaire is that it may encourage some men to seek medical advice. Then they can get their testosterone checked and have a physical examination to help determine whether they are indeed hypogonadal.

Causes of Testosterone Deficiency

As discussed before, hypogonadism is caused when the testicles fail to produce normal levels of testosterone. In one type of hypogonadism, testosterone levels are low, while LH and FSH are elevated. In another, there is not enough secretion of LH and FSH needed to tell the testicles to produce needed testosterone.

Some commonly used medications such as Megace (an appetite stimulant), Nizoral (an anti-fungal agent), Prednisone (an anti-inflammatory corticosteroid) and Tagamet (an antacid) can also lower testosterone production. Illness and aging can cause a decrease in testosterone and/or an increase in sex hormone biding globulin (SHBG). Furthermore, high prolactin hormone levels may suggest a pituitary tumor that may be causing a decrease in testosterone production.

It is important that your doctor measure hormones in the HPGA cascade to diagnose what kind of hypogonadism you have. The most common kind of hypogonadism presents low testosterone with normal or elevated FSH and LH levels, which indicates that your testicles are not responding to the signals of both LH and FSH. This is what is called primary hypogonadism.

There are several reasons that testosterone levels may be low:

- Too much testosterone is being converted into estrogen through theactivity of the aromatase enzyme, and/or the liver is failing to remove excess estrogen. This could be caused by heavy alcohol intake or the effect of some medications on estrogen clearance in the liver.
- Too much free testosterone is being bound by SHBG. This would be especially apparent if a male's total testosterone level is in the high reference range but his free testosterone (unbound) level is low. As previously mentioned, aging and illness increase SHBG.
- The pituitary gland which controls testosterone production through the production of LH, is not secreting enough LH to stimulate production of testosterone by the testicles. In this case, total testosterone would be low.
- The hypothalamus is not functioning properly. LH levels of less than 2 ng/mL suggest a lesion in this part of the HPGA.
- The testicles have lost their ability to produce testosterone, despite adequate amounts of LH. In this case, the level of LH would be high (greater than 10ng/mL) despite a low testosterone level.
- Dehydroepiandrosterone (DHEA) level is abnormally low. DHEA is a hormone produced by the adrenal glands that has a lot of the same benefits as testosterone. It also is a precursor to testosterone in women.

- Disease or infections.
- Street drugs, prescription or over-the-counter medications (more on this later).
- Foods (more on this later).
- Lab error.
- High prolactin levels, which may indicate the presence of a pituitary tumor that impairs production of hormones that tell your testicles to produce testosterone (rare condition but worth mentioning!)
- Defects in genes that affect LH and FSH production.

Diagnosis of Testosterone Deficiency

Lab work will play an important role in diagnosing hypogonadism. Your doctor will likely check your total testosterone and your free testosterone levels. There are some things you should know about these tests, including what they represent and when they should be done.

A "normal" total testosterone scale from most laboratories is generally between 300 and 1,000 ng/dL for men and between 25 and a round 90 ng/dL for women. The normal range from most laboratories for free testosterone usually is between 3.06 and 24 ng/dL for men and between 0.09 and 1.28 ng/dL for women.

As mentioned earlier, free testosterone is not bound to blood carrier proteins, so it is "free" to diffuse readily into cells where it signals them to adjust their activity. Some studies report that free testosterone may be a better indicator for quality of life and lean body mass, but there are some conflicting studies on this issue.

Since aging and illness can increase SHBG, which can attach to testosterone to impair its effectiveness, it becomes more important to test for free testosterone if you are older or being challenged by illness.

Many doctors treat their patients according to hypogonadism symptoms *regardless* of what their testosterone blood levels are. They use optimal ranges of 500 to 1,000 ng/dL for total testosterone and 100 to 200 ng/dL for free testosterone for men and 50 to 100 ng/dL for total testosterone and 1 to 2 ng/dL for free testosterone for women. Table 2 shows the reference ranges for free testosterone according to age in men.

Age-related Decline In Testosterone Levels

Figure 5. Testosterone decreases as we age (Courtesy of Medscape)

As you can see in Figure 5, testosterone decreases as we age. This decline is due to many factors that get in the way of retaining a healthy testosterone blood level. Among them are inflammatory states caused by being over-weight, diet, medications, alcohol and street drug abuse, stress, lack of ade-quate sleep, and problems with how the body uses carbohydrates for energy (due to impaired function of the blood sugar controlling hormone insulin). Some experts also think that our own bodies are slowly turning down their engines to get ready for a slower pace and eventual death. However, many physicians in the aging field have now begun to believe that we can grow older while keeping our strength, sexual function, lean tissue, and cognitive function so that we have more "disability-free" years.

Testosterone levels can vary throughout the day. Young and adult men tend to have higher testosterone levels in the morning than in the evening (see Figure 6). This variation is less evident as men age, however. This fact may explain why it's not uncommon for men to have morning erections.

Some physicians recommend doing hormone testing in the morning on an empty stomach, as many things can affect free testosterone measurements, including diet. Elevated insulin caused by eating carbohydrates, for instance, can increase free testosterone levels by reducing plasma levels of SHBG.

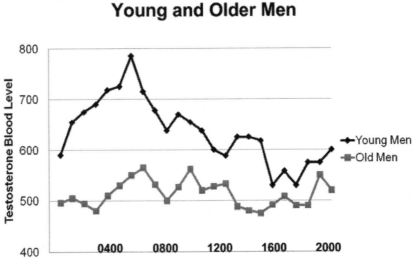

Source: Bremner WJ, Vitiello MV, Prinz PN., *J Clin Endocrinol Metab* 1983;56:1278-1281

Figure 6. Variations in testosterone blood levels during the day for young and older men.

Some doctors tend to test this hormone in the late afternoon since the levels may be lower then. In my opinion, it is not practical to restrict testing of this hormone to early morning times and in a fasting state since intraday fluctuations are not that great in men over 30 and it may be equal to laboratory variability.

Normal values may vary from lab to lab depending on what reference range they use. Your doctor will have your test results in one to two days. Depending on the country, ranges are in nanograms per deciliter (usually in the United States) or nanomoles per liter (Europe and other countries). The conversion factor is:

Testosterone in ng/dL × 0.035 = Testosterone in nanomolars per liter

Table 2. Laboratory Ranges and Codes (courtesy of LabCorp)

Total Testosterone for Males	
Age	
7 months to 9 years	Less than 30 ng/dL (< 1.04 nmol/L)
10–13 years	1–619 ng/dL (0.04–21.48 nmol/L)
14–15 years	100–540 ng/dL (3.47–18.74 nmol/L)
16–19 years	200–970 ng/dL (6.94–33.66 nmol/L)
20–39 years	270–1,080 ng/dL (9.00–37.48 nmol/L)
40–59 years	350–890 ng/dL (12.15–30.88 nmol/ L)
60 years and older	350–720 ng/dL (12.15–24.98 nmol/L)
Reference Intervals for Free Testosterone	
Age	
20–29 years old	9.3–26.5 picograms/mililiter (pg/mL)
30–39 years old	8.7–25.1 pg/mL
40–49 years old	6.8–21.5 pg/mL
50–59 years old	7.2–24.0 pg/mL

-3-

Testosterone Replacement Options

Top Mistakes People Make When Taking Testosterone Replacement Therapy

I have heard of so many mistakes being made by people taking testosterone replacement therapy. Some mistakes seriously impacted their quality of life, or resulted in men stopping testosterone prematurely. Here are a few of the biggest errors I've witnessed:

1. **Using "street sources" of testosterone:** I have met many men whose doctors do not support their use of testosterone, so they buy it on the black market or from some guy at their gyms. This is illegal. Testosterone is classified as a controlled substance under the Anabolic Steroids Control Act of 1990 and has been assigned to Schedule III. It is regulated by the Drug Enforcement Agency (DEA). A doctor can legally prescribe it but it is illegal to use without a prescription. Be aware that the buying or the using of testosterone without a proper prescription may have legal consequences. The use of testosterone and its cousin molecules (anabolic steroids) is illegal in the United States for those without a medical diagnosis that justifies their use (e.g. anemia, wasting, hypogonadism). If after reading this book you still decide to get testosterone in the black market, be beware that you could set up by informants who may alert the DEA of your purchase. Also, importing testosterone even if you have a prescription is not legal. In a nut shell: only use testosterone after a physician gives you a prescription and do not import it from other countries.

    The use of "street" testosterone is also dangerous. No one knows what those products may contain. Some so-called testosterone products may simply contain peanut oil, sesame or grape-seed oil. You also run the risk of exposure to contaminants that could cause infection.

Not having a doctor follow-up your blood work is a sure way to get in trouble! If you have low testosterone, there are hundreds of doctors who will prescribe testosterone replacement therapy (refer to the Appendix section for directories). If you are using testosterone to increase muscle mass or to improve athletic performance even though you have normal testosterone levels, be smart and research all you can. And please, read the information in this book about how stopping testosterone can cause health problems (if you are using black market testosterone, chances are that your source will eventually run out).

2. **Not exploring what testosterone option is best for you**: Since there is an assortment of options for testosterone replacement, it's important that you take the time to really find out what's best for you. Several factors are involved in deciding what would be the best testosterone replacement option for you. Among them are cost, insurance coverage, convenience, preference for daily versus weekly use, lack of time to stick to a strict daily schedule, fears of needles, and physician familiarity of the different products. For instance, some health management organizations (HMOs) programs only pay for testosterone injections since they are the cheapest option. However some men have needle-phobia and dislike weekly or bi-weekly injections that may require them to go see their doctors that frequently (some doctors do not teach their patients to self inject at home). Other men are prescribed daily gels even if their busy lives make it difficult to be perfectly compliant to the daily therapy. Some men without insurance or financial means decide not to seek help since they do not know that there are patient assistance programs set up by manufacturers, or the fact that compounding pharmacies can make cheap gels and creams with a doctor prescription (details on this information is available in the Appedix section). Every testosterone option has advantages and disadvantages that may be more suitable for one person over another, so read the following section on treatment options.

3. **Not using the right dose:** Men who start testosterone need to have their testosterone blood levels rechecked two weeks or one month after they start therapy (depending on the testosterone formulation), right before they administer the corresponding dose for that day or

week. This is critical since these results are essential to deciding if the dose is right for you. Total testosterone blood levels under 500 ng/dL that are not improving your sexual desire and energy should be increased to 500 to 1,000 ng/dL by increasing the frequency of injection or the dose. Some doctors fail to retest after they get a patient started on testosterone since they assume most men respond to 200 mg bi-weekly injections or 5 grams per day of gels. The reality is that many men require higher doses to reach total testosterone levels above mid range of normal. Those men tend to stop testosterone early because they perceive no benefits at "average" doses. Incorrect frequency of injections is a common mistake and is actually worse than not getting treatment at all. See the next sections for more details on this.

4. **Cycling on and off testosterone:** Testosterone replacement is a life-long commitment in most cases. Once you start you should assume that you will stay on it unless you have an unmanageable side effect. Some patients think that "giving the body a break" once every few weeks is a good thing. What they do not know is that during the time that you are taking testosterone, your testicles stop producing it. When you stop replacement therapy you are left with *no* testosterone in your system for weeks while your HPG hormonal axis normalizes. Depression, weight loss, lack of motivation, and loss of sex drive can appear rapidly and with a vengeance. A few men never have their hormonal axis return to normal after stopping testosterone (especially if they were hypogonadal at baseline). Read more details on this in the section entitled "HPGA dysfunction."

5. **Stopping testosterone abruptly due to an unrelated signal:** Some of us may be taking medications for other conditions along with testosterone. Sometimes new medications can increase cholesterol and triglycerides and/or liver enzymes (I call these "signals"). Some doctors prematurely blame testosterone instead of the new medications that someone might have started. I have seen people suffer because of this poor judgment of their doctors. Weeks later, they learn that stopping testosterone did not improve any of these problems but by then they feel tired, depressed, and asexual.

6. **Not knowing how to manage potential side effects:** Luckily, this will not happen to you after you finish reading this book. I know men who stopped testosterone due to swelling in their nipple area, acne,

moodiness, perceived lack of benefit, hair loss, or a prostatic specific antigen (PSA) increase that was due to a prostatic infection. Knowing how to manage these side effects is essential to long-term success. If you know what side effects may occur and how to deal with them, you are less likely to prematurely stop therapy. You may just need to readjust the dose, change the delivery method, or take a medication to counteract the potential problem. Only the best physicians, who do not overreact to a side effect, know how to do this.

7. **Having a life style that is not "testosterone friendly":** If you smoke, drink more than two drinks a day, smoke too much pot, are overweight, do not exercise, do not keep your blood sugar or lipids in control, and do not show up to doctor's appointments, you do not have a testosterone-friendly lifestyle. Studies have shown that these factors may influence your sexual function and long-term health. Excessive alcohol can decrease testosterone. Exercise can increase it if done properly or decrease it if overdone. You can read more about this later in this book.

8. **Not reading or staying "networked" with other patients:** Being in isolation about information makes you a less effective patient. There are online groups of men who discuss testosterone and other issues (see the Resource section). Sharing your experiences and learning from others are keys to being an empowered and proactive patient. It's the only way to maximize the benefits of any therapy you are using. Many of the practical "tricks" that I have learned have been obtained via this method. The collective wisdom of other people with similar issues is more powerful than just relying on everything your doctor tells, or does not tell you. Besides, most doctors treat educated patients a lot better than those who are timid about sharing and asking questions.

9. **Not switching doctors when you have to:** Changing doctors can be difficult, especially if you are not a networked patient who reads a lot about your condition. Many people do not have options and have to see a certain doctor in a health management organization (HMO) setting. But most of us have the option of searching for educated doctors who are not condescending and who treat you as an equal. Your doctor should be your partner in your health and not just an unquestioned authority. Although they are saving lives and have spent hundreds of hours in school and practice to do so, they are human beings who are

exposed to myths and misconceptions similar to ours I have heard the most irrational things from doctors about testosterone replacement that make me question how unfortunate their patients may be. Be sure to do your homework and find a doctor who supports *you* in your search for optimum health. See the Resource section for directories of physicians who are trained in testosterone replacement management.

10. **Poor compliance:** Forgetting when to inject or apply gels is a common complaint. Good time management and reminders are key. Find reminders that work for you. I use Google calendar which can be set up to send me text messages to my phone as reminders. Avoid the yo-yo effect that poor compliance causes! Testosterone replacement is a lifetime and life style commitment that should be explored with care.

Testosterone Formulations

In theory testosterone replacement should approximate the body's own natural production of the hormone. The average male produces 4 to 7 mg of testosterone a day with plasma levels in early morning and lower levels in the evening. Women produce around a 12th of those rates.

Testosterone replacement is usually a life-long commitment. It is a decision that should not be made without a discussion with your health care provider. Starting and stopping testosterone can have negative effects on someone's quality of life (more on this topic later).

There are testosterone replacement products that require daily dosing (orals, buccal, and gels), once a week or two weeks dosing (injections), and once every three- to four-month dosing (long-acting testosterone undecanoate injections (not yet approved in the United States as of 2010) or testosterone pellets).

Males who are hypogonadal can be given continuous testosterone replacement therapy in a wide assortment of ways. These include:

1. Oral capsules
2. Testosterone injections
3. Transdermal (absorbed through the skin) testosterone cream or gel
4. Transdermal testosterone patch
5. Buccal (sublingual and gum adherent)
6. Pellets (that are implanted subcutaneously)

Oral Agents

Oral testosterone formulations are quickly absorbed by the liver and therefore require relatively large doses. Because of the risk of liver toxicity they are rarely prescribed. Do not waste your money or time using oral testosterone. Also, avoid over-the-counter supplements that claim to increase testosterone. Most do *not* increase testosterone for more than a few minutes and can also affect your liver and blood pressure. Oral testosterone also seems to cause larger decreases of the good cholesterol (HDL) than other forms of testosterone therapies.

Chemically unbound testosterone, if taken orally, is immediately deactivated by the liver. Two chemically modified forms of testosterone are available that require several doses a day: methyltestosterone and testosterone undecanoate (not approved in the United States but popular in Canada).

Methyltestosterone

Methyltestosterone is one of the earliest available oral testosterones. Its chemical structure is the hormone testosterone with an added methyl group at the c-17 alpha position of the molecule to slow down its clearance by the liver. The use of oral c-17 alpha methylated testosterone causes toxicity to the liver and is not recommended for testosterone hormone therapy. Brand names around the world include "Metesto," "Methitest," "Testred," "Oreton Methyl," and "Android." These products are responsible for many of the misconceptions that still exist about testosterone replacement due to their liver and lipid problems. The same information is applicable to fluroxymesterone, another oral formulation no longer used in the United States.

Testosterone undecanoate

Testosterone undecanoate is not a c-17 alpha alkylated hormone. Therefore it is considered a safer oral form of testosterone. It is designed to be absorbed through the small intestine into the lymphatic system, and has fewer negative effects on the liver. Brand names around the world for oral testosterone undecanoate include "Andriol," "Androxon," "Understor," "Restandol," and "Restinsol." It is not available in the United States but widely used in Canada and some European countries.

One disadvantage of orally administered undecanoate is that it is eliminated from the body very quickly, usually within three to four hours. Frequent administration is necessary—usually from three to six capsules a day, which makes it impractical for most men with busy lives.

> PERSONAL COMMENT: I've never used oral testosterones and I never will. Other formulations are so much more user-friendly.

Intramuscular Injections

The most common testosterone replacement used by men worldwide is intramuscular testosterone injection. It's also the oldest and most economical way to increase blood levels of testosterone. This most cost effective option is usually covered by insurance programs and community clinics.

The two most common esters, testosterone cypionate and testosterone enanthate, are both generic medications in the United States. They are given at a weekly dose of about 100 to 200 mg a week (or 200 to 300 mg every two weeks).

Behre HM et al. In: *Testosterone: Action, Deficiency, Substitution.* Berlin, Germany: Springer-Verlag; 1998:329-348

Figure 7. Yo-yo effect of peaks and valleys when injecting testosterone.

Currently, a 10 ml bottle of 200 mg/ml (2000 total milligrams per bottle) of testosterone cypionate obtained in U.S. pharmacies cost around $115. For a dose of 200 mg every two weeks (or 100 mg per week), the monthly cost for this injections would be $23, plus the cost of syringes. Some physicians have patients come to their office for injections and others empower their patients to do so at home. A minority of physicians charges a fee for the office visit when you come for an injection, which can increase your costs.

When you get a prescription for any testosterone ester, make sure that it is for a 10-ml vial, not 1-ml vial. In the U.S., 1-ml vials are available but they are usually more expensive and not very practical. Many physicians will write an open-ended prescription that will look like this:

1. *Testosterone Cypionate (or Depo Testosterone), 10 ml, 200mg/ml, #1, as directed, 1 refill*

Others will write:

2. *Testosterone Cypionate, 10 ml, 200 mg/ml, #1, 200 mg q 2 weeks, 1 refill*

Or

3. *Tetsosterone Cypionate , 10 ml, 200 mg/ml #1, 100 mg q 1 week, 1 refill*

Be sure your physician gives you a more flexible prescription that reads like my first example. This type of prescription will provide room for you to adjust the dosage during the first two months as well as get a refill whenever you need it.

Optimum testosterone doses can range from 100 mg to 300 mg a week but it is practically impossible to predict an individual's response. Giving yourself a little room for adjustment keeps you from running out of testosterone if your insurance company denies your next refill because they think it's too early. Of course, your physician has to ensure that your dose is adjusted based on your total or free testosterone blood levels.

When using injectable testosterone, your doctor will wantto measure your total blood testosterone levels right before your next injection after the first month (it takes a while for the blood levels to stabilize). If testosterone is >700 ng/dl (24.5 nmol/liter) or <350 ng/dl (12.3 nmol/liter), adjust dose or frequency. Some men need to have levels above 500 ng/dl to experience any of the expected sexual function benefits. It is important to be honest about your answers to questions from your doctor about your sexual performance.

A dose for women is anywhere from 2.4 to 20 mg/week but because it is difficult to inject such low doses and because of the risk of masculinization (growth or facial hair, deepening of the voice, and growth of clitoris), many doctors prefer low dose creams to treat women. Compounding pharmacies like Women's International Pharmacy can guide doctors on how to test and prescribe testosterone gels to women. Their website is womensinterna-tional.com.   There is no commercially available FDA-approved testosterone therapy for women in the United States as of 2010, but two options may be approved in 2011. However, many doctors can legally prescribe testosterone to women in an off-label manner. Many are reluctant to prescribe any hormones to women since the discouraging results from female hormone replacement in women showed increased cardiovascular risk in women. For a great articles and books on women and hormones, I highly recommend Dr Susan Rako's page: www.susanrako. com/workshop.htm

There are several types of testosterone esters: testosterone cypionate, enanthate, propionate, or undecanoate. Outside the United States, there is a product with a combination of the first three esters that is called Sustanon 250 (250 mg of a mixture of cypionate, enanthate, and propionate). Since every ester may have slightly different blood decay after administration, it is speculated that this combination may allow better distribution of testosterone blood levels in 14 days. Sustanon is not available in the United States but compounding pharmacies may customize similar formulations.

Testosterone cypionate, enanthate, or any other ester is injected slowly into the muscle of the buttock where it forms a reservoir of the hormone. Then testosterone is gradually released from the reservoir into the blood stream. There is usually a peak concentration in the blood within the first two days and then a gradual decrease to baseline. Everyone is different and the rate of decrease of blood levels tends to change depending on body weight, fat content, activity level, medications, illness, and liver metabolism.

There is also a new, long-acting product being reviewed by the FDA in the United States called Aveed (Nebido is the brand name worldwide) that contains testosterone undecanoate, which is injected at a dose of 1,000 mg in Europe (the FDA may not allow that large of a dose in one injection, though) and which produces sustained total testosterone levels above 400 nanograms/dl in four to five months. Water-based "suspensions" are also available but they are shorter acting and tend to hurt more when injected, so they are not often used.

Injections have the advantage of once-per-week (or every two weeks) administration, so it may be a more acceptable option for men who do not want to deal with the daily administration typically needed with gels. However there are concerns about their "peak-and-valleys" testosterone blood level patterns.

As you can see in Figures 7 and 8, 200 mg testosterone injections currently used in the United States produce an unnaturally high blood testosterone level during the initial few days after an injection. Then the blood level drops off each day and falls to baseline in about 10 days. This method does not effectively deliver sustained normal blood levels of testosterone or mimic the natural daily pattern of testosterone release as well as other treatment options. There is a concern that some men using 200 mg of testosterone cypionate every two weeks may have low levels of testosterone by day 10, so they spend four days with low testosterone before their next injection.

Testosterone Blood Levels After a 200 mg Injection

Figure 8 Blood testosterone concentration curve after a 200 mg injection of testosterone cypionate.

Your doctor should re-check your testosterone level after one month (after steady state occurs) right before the next injection. This testing schedule allows him to see whether normal levels are still present when you reach your lowest testosterone blood level. If serum total testosterone level is more than 1000 ng/dL or less than 500 ng/dL right before the next dose, he can adjust the dose or the frequency accordingly.

Due to testosterone's effect as a stimulant of red blood cell production, injections produce unusually strong stimulation during the first peak days. This appears to increase the potential for elevated hemoglobin and hematocrit indicating that you have too many red blood cells. These can increase your cardiovascular risks. Creams, gels, and patches appear to be less likely to produce this side effect, though study results are conflicting.

Anecdotally I hear that injections promote elevations in blood pressure more than creams, gel, and patches. It also appears that the effect on brain chemistry and the nervous system that might promote increased assertiveness can be stronger with injections. There will be more discussion on this subject later. But I would love to see head-to-head comparison studies between testosterone injections and gels, since none have been performed to date. Hopefully, with the potential approval of Aveed in the future, its manufacturer would be compelled to do such a study to convince insurance companies that their product may be more cost effective and less problematic than the daily gels currently approved in the United States (Androgel and Testim).

I have met some men that have switched from injections to gels and then eventually switch back to injections. It seems that they need the higher level of overall metabolic stimulation that injectable testosterone provides. Usually,those men also say they feel very little improvement with the use of gels or creams. They also usually prefer the convenience of an injection every one or two weeks to the daily administration of a gel. And, unlike gels, injections have no potential risk of transferring testosterone through hugging other people.

Injectable testosterone has also shown to increase blood levels of testosterone and DHT in proportion with the dose. But gels seem to increase DHT a lot more than the expected increase due to higher testosterone, so some men with benign prostatic inflammation may prefer injections than gels.

As you can see, there is no one-size-fits-all approach that works for everyone. Blank statements about one option being better than other have to be done in the context of other factors that gone beyond the obvious.

It is important to follow a strict injection procedure (for helpful tips, see the section on How to Inject Testosterone Safely). Some men report soreness in the injection area and experience coughing spells after injecting. Some have got infections in the injection site due to unsanitary techniques!

Commonly Used Injectable Esters for Testosterone Replacement Therapy

Testosterone esters are modifications made to the testosterone molecule to increase the time the liver breaks it down, so that you do not have to inject every day. Esters consist of the actual testosterone molecule, with a carbon chain attached to it. This carbon chain controls something called the partition co-efficient, which translates into how soluble the drug will be once in the bloodstream. Also, the larger the carbon chain, the longer the ester, the less soluble the drug is in water, and the longer it stays in your body. Also, additions to the basic testosterone molecule make it harder for the liver to break it down, which also increases the time testosterone stays in your system (a good thing since we do not want to deal with injections too frequently).

There are several types of testosterone esters: testosterone cypionate, enanthate, propionate, or undecanoate. Outside the United States, there is a product with a combination of the first three esters that is called Sustanon 250 (250 mg of a mixture of cypionate, enanthate, and propionate). Since every ester may have slightly different blood level decay after administration, it is speculated that this combination may allow better distribution of testosterone blood levels in 14 days. Sustanon is not available in the United States but compounding pharmacies may customize similar formulations.

Testosterone cypionate, enanthate, or other ester is injected slowly into the muscle of the buttock where it forms a reservoir of the hormone. Then testosterone is gradually released from the reservoir into the blood stream. There is usually a peak concentration in the blood within the first two days and then a gradual decrease to baseline. Everyone is different and the rate of decrease of blood levels tends to change depending on body weight, fat content, activity level, medications, illness, and liver metabolism.

Testosterone Enanthate

Testosterone enanthate is one of the main forms of testosterone prescribed to men in the United States. It is a slow-acting ester, with a release time between 8 and 10 days. The name brand of testosterone enanthate available in the United States is called "Delatestryl," which is suspended in sesame oil. Testosterone enanthate is typically injected once every week to once every two weeks. Generic testosterone enanthate can also be obtained through a compounding pharmacy; such pharmacies can mix the enanthate in either sesame, grapeseed or cottonseed oil. Some mix different esters for patients who think this will give better blood leveldistribution, although no studies have been done in the United States using ester blends.

For more details about this product, refer to the Appendix section for the package insert. Package inserts are required by the FDA to be provided with every product when you pick it up at the pharmacy. They are also required when magazine ads or promotional materials are provided on products. That is why I thought it would be a good idea to include a package insert on an injectable and a gel at the end of this book. Every patient should read package inserts of every medication they take, but keeping in mind that a lot of the side effects listed are not common and only happen in special circumstances. But it does not hurt to know them just in case!

Testosterone cypionate

Testosterone cypionate is the other main injectable form of testosterone prescribed to men in the United States. It is a slow-acting ester with a release time of 8 to 10 days, similar to that of enanthate. The name brand available in the United States is called "Depo-Testosterone," which is suspended in cottonseed oil. Testosterone cypionate is typically injected anywhere from once every week to once every two weeks. Some doctors like to prescribe 300 mg every three weeks, but I believe that really accentuates the peaks and valleys of testosterone blood levels a lot more than the most commonly used dose of 100 or 200 mg every two weeks. Cheaper generic testosterone cypionate can also be obtained through a compounding pharmacy which can mix it in either sesame, grapeseed or cotton seed oil.

Sustanon 100 or 250

"Sustanon" is the brand name for two formulas of injectable testosterone that contain a blend of esters. "Sustanon 100" contains 100 mg of three testosterone esters: testosterone propionate, testosterone phenylpropionate, and testosterone isocaproate. "Sustanon 250" contains a total of 250 mg of four testosterone esters: testosterone propionate, testosterone phenylpropionate, testosterone isocaproate, and testosterone decanoate. Both formulas feature fast-acting and slow-acting esters, and can be injected anywhere from once every week to once every four weeks. Sustanon is prescribed outside the United States, but a formulation similar to it can be compounded legally by compounding pharmacies since all of its esters are available in the United States.

Other Injectable Esters of Testosterone

Testosterone propionate

Testosterone propionate is a fast-acting ester with a release time of three to four days. To keep blood levels from fluctuating greatly, propionate is usually injected from one to three times a week. It is for this reason that it is not usually prescribed that much. Some users also report that propionate is a more painful injection, with swelling and noticeable pain around the injection site.

Testosterone phenylpropionate

Testosterone phenylpropionate is a slow-acting ester, with a release time of one to three weeks. A popular name brand for T-phenylpropionate is "Testolent." Testosterone phenylpropionate is also one of the components of Sustanon.

Testosterone Undecanoate

Testosterone undecanoate injections are known as the brand name Nebido around the world. In the United States it will be called Aveed. Aveed is currently under review for approval by the FDA. This ester may stay longer in your system so that less frequent injections may be needed. The injection is usually given once every 10 to 14 weeks, though the frequency will depend on your individual testosterone levels. After your first injection you may be asked to come back for another injection at week six. The company claims that only five injections a year are needed (compare to.

In an open-label study which enrolled 130 hypogonadal men with blood total testosterone levels below 300 ng/dL at study entry, Aveed was dosed as an intramuscular injection (750 mg) at baseline, at week four, and then every 10 weeks throughout the remainder of the 21-month study. Approximately 70 percent of patients completed all injections and 94 percent of them had total testosterone from 300 to 1,000 nanograms/ml through the entire study.

After Nebido was approved in Europe a small number of European patients experienced respiratory symptoms immediately following an intramuscular injection of 1000 mg in a 4 cc injection volume, (versus the 750 mg, 3 cc injection volume used in the United States). The makers of Nebido believe, and the FDA concurs, that the reaction is likely the result of a small amount of the oily solution immediately entering the vascular system from the injection site. This known yet uncommon complication of oil-based depot injections may be related to inappropriate injection technique or site.

The problem is characterized by short-term reactions involving an urge to cough or a shortness of breath. In some rare cases the reaction had been classified as serious or the patient had experienced other symptoms such as dizziness, flushing or fainting. In U.S. clinical trials of Nebido 750 mg (3 cc injection volume), the proposed dose in the U.S., there was a single, mild, non-serious case of oil-based coughing.

Figure 9. Two bottles of testosterone cypionate, the most commonly used injectable in the United States

The U.S. manufacturer, Endo Pharmaceuticals, is gathering data to address concerns about the respiratory symptoms. It is not known how much longer it will take the get this product approved in the United States as of June 2010. And even if it gets approved, it may not be widely available for people to buy through private health insurance if the company decides to price it as high as gels.

PERSONAL COMMENT: I have used testosterone enanthate, cypionate, and Sustanon 250. I cannot say I can tell the difference in the way I felt. I also tried one injection of Nebido in Mexico. After a big injection of the recommended dose of 1,000 mg, my testosterone blood levels remained above 450 ng/ml for four and a half months; my mood and stamina remained very good throughout. It was nice not having to worry about remembering to inject every two weeks.

How to Inject Testosterone Safely

Some men prefer testosterone injections because of the convenient dosing and/or they report feeling much better when using injections versus gels. Sometimes their insurance companies only pay for injections. Men without health insurance also tend to use injections since they are a lot cheaper than gels. If your doctor empowers you to self-inject at home, it will be more convenient and possible cheaper (some physicians charge for the office visit). I tell men that they can always switch from gels to injections and vice versa depending on what they learn as they optimize their testosterone replacement.

So you've decided to go with injectable testosterone. Your decision may arise out of your realization that you won't remember to make daily use of the gels. It may have made the choice because your insurance company refuses to pay for anthing but the injectable. If your doctor is letting you self-inject there are some things for you to know:

- **Keep it safe**. Sharing used needles with another person is a definite NO. No, no and no! And this goes for the syringes too. You can contract all kinds of diseases including hepatitis B and C, and HIV. Doctors give you a prescription for syringes and needles for a reason. There is no need to risk ruining your health. Don't even think about re-using your own syringes and needles. Unclean needles and syringes can cause infections. Buy a "sharps" container and put your used needles and syringes in it. These containers are available at most pharmacies. Those using underground testosterone usually have the most difficult time trying to find syringes since pharmacies won't provide supplies without a prescription.

- **Keep it moving**. Try not to inject into the exact same area more than twice a month. Vigorously massage the area after you've injected. This helps reduce pain.
- **Keep it clean**. Wash your hands before starting. Clean the area to be injected using an alcohol swab. Clean the top of the testosterone vial with an alcohol swab before you insert the needle to draw the product. The alcohol swabs are available at most pharmacies and do not require a prescription.
- **Keep it sharp**. Use a new needle every time. I personally like using smaller gauge needles, which are bigger in size (18 gauge, 1 inch), to draw the testosterone from the bottle. I then use a new larger gauge needle, which is smaller in size (23 gauge, 1 inch) when injecting. The reason for this is that after a needle is used once, it loses its sharpness. Injections with dull needles hurt a lot more. I ask the pharmacist to sell me several 18 gauge needles without syringes for drawing the testosterone, plus the same number of 23 gauge, 1 inch, 3 ml syringes.
- What to look for before injecting.
  - **Expiration dates**
    - Check the expiry dates of every product.
  - **Waste**
    - Make sure that contaminated waste is disposed of safely. Ask your pharmacist to sell you a plastic sharps container.
  - **Materials needed**
    - Vial with required testosterone, 20-23 gauge syringe with a capacity of 3 ml and a needle length of 1-1.5 inches, an extra 18 gauge needle for drawing testosterone into syringe, two alcohol swabs.

Guide to Injecting Testosterone (courtesy of Forge.org):

1. Wash your hands (with a disinfectant/anti-bacterial soap).
2. Layout your vial of testosterone, needle(s) and/or syringe, alcohol wipes, and tissue on a clean surface (e.g. a clean towel, paper towel, etc).
3. Sit down and get comfy.
4. Secure the lure-lock on the fit on the syringe.
5. Unseat/loosen the cap from the needle. Leave the cap on loose until ready to draw the testosterone. Remember not to touch the needle!

6. Wipe off the "nipple" on the top of the vial with an alcohol wipe.

7. Remove the cap of the needle without touching the needle or the needle touching anything. Draw around 1 cc of air into the syringe by pulling back on the plunger.

8. Up-end the testosterone vial.

9. Insert the needle through the center of the neoprene nipple.

10. With the needle tip immersed *IN the* fluid, slowly depress the plunger, pushing all of the air into the oil (you'll see the bubbles).

11. After all the air is out of the syringe, slowly pull back on the plunger until the proper amount of testosterone is drawn into the syringe. (Not everyone's dosage is the same. Check your prescription or consult with your physician or pharmacist for the correct amount. Some will inject more than 1 cc, some less.)

12. You may need to "pump" the plunger to get a complete fill. As long as you don't remove the needle, you can let the fluid go in and out as much as needed.

13. When you have the correct amount in the syringe, gently pull the needle out of the vial.

14. Draw a small amount of air into the syringe—one very small bubble.

15. Slip the needle back into the cap if you want to take a break before injecting. (It's really important not to touch the needle itself at any point.)

16. Pick an injection site on your thigh or buttocks. You'll want to alternate sites, so remember which site you last injected. For your thigh, target the spot by placing one hand just about at your knee and the other at your hip—the area in between is pretty much fair game. The best area is the outer part of the quad, so stay to the outside of the midline of your thigh, but not too far to the outside/underside. The buttocks is slightly more tricky—both to reach and to isolate the exact spot. Talk to your physician or nurse about the exact location.

17. Clean the injection site with an alcohol wipe. Wipe in a circular motion, to a circumference of about two inches surrounding the injection site. Allow the skin to dry to prevent the alcohol from being introduced into the muscle as the needle is inserted, causing pain or burning. Remember not to touch the area just cleansed with the alcohol wipe.

18. Uncap the needle—remember not to touch the needle or the swabbed area on your thigh. The air bubble should be near the plunger end of the syringe.

19. Go to it and stick it in! Fast or slow, either is fine. Pierce the skin at a 90 degree angle. It must go through the subcutaneous tissue/fatty tissue and deep into the muscle.

20. If using a 1" needle, stop about 1/8" from the base; if using a 1.5" needle, stop about 1/4" from the base. (This is true for average- sized bodies. Talk with your physician about the appropriate needle length for your body.)

21. After the needle has been inserted, aspirate by holding the barrel of the syringe steady with your non dominant hand and by pulling back on the plunger with your dominant hand. You'll see some air bubbles in the testosterone. If there's just air/clear fluid—no blood—then it's ok to proceed. If there is blood, either push the needle in or pull the needle back a little and pull back on the plunger again, or pull the needle out and start over.

22. Holding the syringe steady, inject the testosterone steadily and slowly by depressing the plunger until all of the testosterone is injected. The air bubble in the syringe should follow the testosterone and will "pack" the testosterone down into your muscle. There will be a slight a "pop" as the bubble leaves the syringe.

23. Pull the needle out—again, slow or fast depending upon your preference. (I think it's usually best to pull out slow—sounds dirty, doesn't it?!) Sometimes the injection site may bleed a little when you withdraw the needle, just be prepared to apply some gentle pressure with some clean tissue(s).

24. Slide the needle back into the cap. (Remember DO NOT reseat the cap by pressing the tip of the cap towards the needle's point.)

25. Dispose of your needles properly in what is known as a sharps container (i.e., a needle disposal container).

Once you inject a few times, you should lose begin to lose your fear of injecting. You can also have your partner or good friend inject you if you do not feel comfortable doing so. Your doctor's medical staff can help you develop your technique.

PERSONAL COMMENT: I think I have great injection technique but I have experienced the post-injection cough. It is a strange feeling compared to inhaling very cold air that makes you cough and feel out of breath for a few minutes. This probably has happened to me

only five times in 16 years of testosterone use When it has happened
I find that breathing quickly into a paper bag helps it go away faster.
Honestly, I cannot tell you if I used a different injection site since I
always use the upper buttock area close to my hip.

For an update on injection techniques, please visit my web site
TestosteroneWisdom.com

Transdermal Systems

Transdermal gels (Androgel, Testim)

As shown in Figure 10, creams and gels may provide lower and more sustained concentrations of testosterone in the blood without the "yo-yo" effect that injections can cause. Testosterone gets absorbed through the skin
in a once or twice daily use.

The best application areas for the gel include the stomach, shoulders,
the inner thighs, and the pectorals. Be aware that some people complain
about dark hair growth where the cream or gel is applied, especially if one
site is used over and over again without rotation

**Mean Steady-State Testosterone
Concentrations in Patients Receiving AndroGel®**

Day 90

Figure 10 Testosterone blood levels are more stable on testosterone gels

As mentioned if you use testosterone this way, it can rub off onto a female partner or children when you hug them. So, it is important that this is kept in mind.

I think that its application on the back of the legs may help avoid this potential transfer of testosterone to other people. Most testosterone in gels and creams gets absorbed in the first one to two hours, but some residual testosterone may still be present after a few hours.

Androgel packets

Testim tubes

Androgel pump for higher doses

Not to scale

Figure 11 Commercially available testosterone gels in the United States

Topical testosterone products represent approximately 65.6 percent of the total number of testosterone prescriptions dispensed between 2000 and November 2008, according to the FDA. Two prescription-based commercial testosterone gels are available in the United States: Androgel,approved by the FDA in February 2000, and Testim, approved in October 2002 (See Figure 11). Approximately 1.4 million prescriptions were dispensed for Androgel and 400,000 prescriptions were dispensed for Testim in 2008. The majority of prescriptions for Androgel are dispensed to adult males 50 to 59 years of age.

Both gels are colorless and evaporate quickly after being applied to the abdomen, shoulders, or arms. Androgel and Testim come in three dose levels (2.5 g, 5 g,and 10 g with 1 percent testosterone each). Ten percent of the applied testosterone is absorbed into the blood stream through the skin. The usual starting dose is a packet of 5 g a day.

Androgel also comes in a pump that allows for higher dosing for those men who do not reach normal testosterone levels with the available gels. Each pump container is capable of dispensing 75 grams or 60 metered 1.25-gram doses. The starting dose of 5 grams a day requires four pump squirts. Many men require up to 10 grams per day to reach total testosterone blood levels above 500 ng/ml. This makes for eight squirts a day of Androgel. For some, that is a lot of volume to spread on the body. Luckily these gels dry up fast and leave little to no residue.

Auxilium, the maker of Testim, claims that their gel has a slightly better absorption rate than Androgel; however, many men do not like its slight soapy smell (Androgel has none).

Androgel and Testim are usually covered by insurance. Their monthly cost is around US$700 a month, with insurance copays ranging from US$20 to US$50 a month. A patient assistance program has been set up by both companies to provide free drug to low-income patients with no insurance (read the resource section in this book for additional information).

At the time of writing this book, some companies were getting ready to manufacture generic testosterone gels which may provide a cheaper alternative.

Regardless of which gel you use, make sure your doctor re-checks your blood levels after two weeks to see whether you need to readjust the dose.

Figure 12 shows the areas where gels are usually applied. Testosterone gels should be applied to clean, dry skin. Do not apply to the testicular area since this has been shown to increase DHT conversion.

Application sites should be allowed to dry for a few minutes before dressing. Hands should be washed thoroughly with soap and water after application. In order to prevent transfer of testosterone to another person, clothing should be worn to cover the application sites. If a direct skin-to-skin contact with another person is anticipated, the application sites should be washed thoroughly with soap and water. Users should wait at least two hours after applying before showering or swimming; for optimal absorption, it may be best to wait five to six hours.

Men who may carry babies should be extra careful to avoid skin-to-skin contact after applying the gel since testosterone exposure in babies may have negative effects on the baby's growth. This fact was included in a recent label change for both Testim and Androgel described in the FDA web site: "Since the initial marketing approval of testosterone gel in 2000 to May 2009, FDA's Adverse Event Reporting System (AERS) received 20 reports (18 U.S. and 2 non-U.S.) describing adverse events in children who were exposed to testosterone gel that was used by another person (referred to as 'secondary exposure'). The adverse events reported in these children included one or more of the following signs or symptoms: enlargement of the penis or clitoris, premature development of pubic hair, advanced bone age, increased self-stimulation, libido, erections, and aggressive behavior. An increased testosterone level was reported in more than half of these cases. The children ranged in age from 9 months to 7 years. Three of the 20 cases are described in the medical literature." Be careful not to come in contact with another person during first 4 hours of administration.

- **Abdomen**
- **Shoulders**
- **Upper arms**

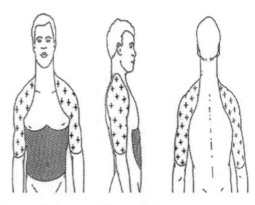

Figure 12 Body areas where gels are usually applied

Compounded creams and gels

Compounded creams and gels can be mixed by compounding pharmacies, and are similar in dosing, application, and precautions to what is described above for Androgel and Testim. There are various qualities of creams and gels made by compounding pharmacies around the United States, and some of the poorer quality products are gunky and flake off after they dry. Be sure to buy from a reputable pharmacy.

The best gels are clear and basically disappear shortly after application. Most men prefer alcohol-based gels, which absorb through the skin better than water-based gels. Creams should not be greasy and should resemble good moisturizing creams. Many compounding pharmacies make cheaper gels and creams with higher testosterone concentrations (2 to 10 percent) for men who do not respond to the commercially available 1 percent testosterone gel products (Testim or Androgel).

Some doctors do not feel comfortable prescribing gels from compounding pharmacies since they worry about quality control. There is also concern that higher concentration gels may induce more DHT conversion, which may cause more prostatic hyperplasia (inflammation) causing urinary flow restrictions especially in older men. Also, higher DHT can cause acne and hair loss.

There are many compounding pharmacies around the United States. Here are some compounding pharmacies with competitive prices that I have used:

- APS Pharmacy. 888-547-2654. APSMeds.com.
- The Compounding Shop. 866-792-6731. GotoCompoundingShop.com.
- College Pharmacy. 800-888-9358.: collegepharmacy.com.
- GBTRx Pharmacy. Phone 866-422-7210. GBTRX.com.

You can also Google the key words: "compounding pharmacy" and your zip code to find compounding pharmacies close to you. Compounding pharmacies ship across state lines, so it is not imperative that you have one in your area. They do not typically take insurance, so you have to request reimbursement from your insurance company. Your doctor has to be willing to call or fax a prescription to the pharmacy for you to order any testosterone products. The compounding pharmacy will need your credit card before shipping the product to you, so make sure you call them to set that up.

Most compounded testosterone gels of 1 to 10 percent concentrations can range between US$17 and US$70 a month so it's worth calling around for price comparisons. Your doctor may have an established relationship with a local compounding pharmacy, so be sure to ask. As mentioned before, some doctors have trust issues with compounding pharmacies' quality control and ask to see their certificates to prove that they have proper quality control standards.

There are two main advantages of using compounding pharmacies for testosterone gel or cream. The first is cost: until a generic version of the gel is available, compounded gel will usually be the cheaper alternative.

The second is customization: your doctor can write a prescription of varying concentration for gels or creams. I have used gels containing 5 and 10 percent testosterone with great results. Of course the volume needed is lower when the concentration increases. Some researchers believe that higher concentration gels tend to increase DHT levels more strongly than the regular 1 percent gels. However many men need more than the usual amount of Testim or Androgel and do not want to smear their bodies with lots of gel, so 5 percent gels may be an option for them.

Most compounding pharmacies dispense the creams in "Topi-Click" (see Figure 13) that are better (typically) than the pre-loaded syringes they are usually supplied in. The Topi-Click is more like a "deodorant stick" which can be more convenient and better looking than the bigger syringes.

Compounded Testosterone- TopiClick Applicator

Some compounding pharmacies: apsmeds.com, gotocompoundingshop.com, gbtrx.com. There should be one in your area (do a google search)

Figure 13 TopiClick Applicator for a compounded testosterone cream

PERSONAL COMMENT: I tried both Androgel and Testim for a few weeks. Both were effective but I admit to having a little sticker shock ($260 to $600 per month depending on dose, if not paid by insurance). Testim had a soapy smell that I didn't particulary like, but some women gave me compliments on my "cologne." I did like the large pump dispenser for Androgel since I could adjust the dosage if needed (I needed 10 grams of gel a day. Most doctors start you at 5 grams per day). I am currently using a testosterone gel/cream formulation with 5 percent testosterone. The prescription is written like this: *Testosterone gel/cream 5 percent 30 mL in Topi-Click, 1 mL a day.* I find the Topi-Click container to be a very easy way to administer the daily dose. You can also order the gel in a large graduated plastic syringe if you want to precise on your dose).

Transdermal patches

Another option for testosterone replacement therapy is a testosterone patch such as Testoderm or Androderm. For many men two 5-mg patches will bring them into the effective mid-range (500 ng/dL and above) of the testosterone blood test. The most frequent complaint with the patch is skin irritation at the application site. Some won't care for the potential of an unwanted "disclosure" since the patch can be visible to anyone who may see you without clothes. You also run the risk of having the patch fall off after sweating or bathing.

Androderm

Androderm comes in two doses: A 2.5 mg/patch and a 5.0 mg/patch. The actual amount of testosterone in the 2.5 mg patch is really 12.2 mg, while in the 5.0 mg patch it is 24.3 mg. Similar to what happens with the gel, much of the testosterone in the patch will not be absorbed into your system. So the aim of the 2.5 mg patch is to get 2.5 mg of testosterone successfully into the blood stream each day. It is possible to absorb slightly more or slightly less than the 2.5 mg patch's ideal dosage (this applies to the 5.0 mg patch as well). Most men need not one but two patches of 5 mg each to attain total testosterone blood levels above 500 ng/dL.

Androderm patches are usually applied on the back, abdomen, thighs, or upper arms. Because the active area of the patch is covered, you can enjoy some worry-free skin contact with your partner. As with any form of testosterone, your blood level will need to be checked by your doctor to determine your dosage. Since dosages vary between 2.5 and 10 mg daily, this may require one or more patches.

It seems from the data that Androderm does not raise DHT or estrogen levels too much, so this may be an advantage for this option.

PERSONAL COMMENT: I have used Androderm and I have to say that I was not very fond of this product. I felt kind of exposed when I was naked, you know what I mean? I didn't want to have to talk about testosterone replacement therapy just when things were getting interesting. Some countries and public clinics provide only Androderm; it is a good option I would not discourage anyone from using it.

Testoderm TTS

Testoderm was first introduced as a patch that you would have to apply to the scrotum (testicular sack) after shaving it. For obvious reasons, it was not very practical and discreet (imagine explaining to any sexual partners what that patch is doing there and that you are not injured as it may seem!). It also showed large increases in DHT since the scrotum tissue seems to facilitate the conversion of testosterone into DHT. For this reason a new non-scrotal patch was developed. Testoderm TTS patches are available in two doses: 4.0 and 6.0 mg/patch. As with Androderm, the actual amount of testosterone in these patches is greater than the listed dose because much of the testosterone will not be absorbed.

Testoderm TTS patches are usually applied on the back, abdomen, thighs, or upper arms. Since the patch is covered, like the Androderm you don't have to worry about transferring the testosterone through skin contact with a partner. Dosages will vary between 4.0 and 10 mg daily requiring one or more patches. Again, your testosterone level will need to be checked by your doctor to determine your dose. Anecdotally Testoderm TTS seems to increase DHT levels more than most other options in the market, although a study showed constant testosterone/DHT ratios, meaning that both values increased in the same proportion.

Testosterone Pellets (Testopel or compounded pellets)

One other option for testosterone replacement therapy are pellets. These are small, sterile cylinders about the size of a grain of rice that are produced by compressing medicated powders. A doctor implants these pellets underneath the skin in the upper buttock area by the hip. They can be used whenever a prolonged continuous absorption of hormones is desired. Men who have problems remembering daily applications, who are afraid of needles, or that travel a lot, may find this option a very practical one.

Men receiving the pellet implants enjoy the convenience of not having to worry about daily dosing normally or weekly injections associated with other delivery systems. Testosterone implants have been around for many years, but many doctors shy away from for several reasons: Doctors need special training to learn the insertion technique; it is difficult to determine the optimal initial number of pellets and is inconvenient to insert addition pellets if needed; the risks of infections in the insertion site. Some users have reported problems with the pellets working their way out from under the skin (called extrusion).

Doctors can charge for the pellets (sold only to doctors), for the procedure, and all blood tests required, so pellets can be a good source of income.

The Testopel pellet—the only one approved by the FDA—contains 75 mg of testosterone. Depending on your body weight and metabolism, and pellet dose, 6–14 pellets are inserted in one procedure. The insertion of the pellets is quick and usually done using a local anesthetic. Pellets typically last 3–4 months. Most patients return to work the day of or the day after implantation, but are advised to avoid bending or vigorous physical activity during this time. Note: I got pellets implanted and flew back home for 2 hours an hour after the procedure and I had no problems.

Some compounding pharmacies can also make testosterone pellets, though it is difficult to determine how effective they are. Compounded pellets can vary from 75 mg to 200 mg a pellet.

Medicaid reimburses $67.50 per pellet, and a 200-pound man usually needs 10-12 pellets to reach adequate blood levels, even though Testopel's package insert recommends 6 pellets. I have talked to some men that did not have insurance and both paid around $1,000 as a total cost for the pellets and doctor's fees. If this therapy is effective for four months, then the cost amounts to $250 a month. Several insurance companies do not reimburse for the pellets, but many are starting to. Medicare pays for them.

I know I'm sounding like a broken record, but remember that it is critical to be monitored so that you know how well this therapy is working.

There is very little data on DHT or estrogen conversion of pellets, but it is speculated that they tend to have the fewest problems in that area for men.

Some doctors are using pellets in an off-label manner in women with low testosterone.

PERSONAL COMMENT: I have used Testopel with great results. Twelve pellets were inserted under the skin of my upper buttocksarea. My total testosterone went up from 350 to 650, and it stayed over 500 for three and half months. It was so great not having to worry about remembering to inject every week or apply gel every day. The tiny pellets were not noticeable to the naked eye after the procedure and disappeared after four months. Pellets are definitely an option to consider if you cannot adhere to daily gels or bi-weekly injections. Some doctors are better than others at inserting them and at getting insurance to pay for this option. A big "thank you" to Dr. Richard Cavender in Ohio who did a great job inserting my pellets quickly and painlessly (www.na-healthassoc.com). He has a comprehensive and pretty amazing wellness clinic with fancy computerized exercise equipment, nutritionists, and a whole gamut of wellness services. Definitely ahead of his time! I understand that he trains physicians on proper pellet insertion techniques.

Sublingual/buccal testosterone

Believe it or not there are yet more options. The sublingual and buccal testosterone forms work by placing either a dissolving tablet under your tongue (sublingual) or a tablet against the surface of the gums (buccal). It is different from an oral delivery in that very little of the substance is swallowed, avoiding potential liver toxicity.

Sublingual

Sublingual testosterone can be obtained through compounding pharmacies as flavored, dissolvable tablets.

Usually 15 mg twice a day will bring total testosterone levels to over 500 ng/dL. Some men may need only once a day dosing. It is still good to check your testosterone blood levels two weeks after daily use to see whether the dose is right for you. It is claimed that no liver toxicities are associated with this option. Some men report a short-term boost in testosterone that may help with arousal right before sex.

PERSONAL COMMENT: GBTRX.com, a compounding pharmacy, has a good mint-tasting product that I have tried. I experienced no increase in my liver enzymes. It's twice a day application was not practical for my busy lifestyle however.

Buccal

In 2003, the FDA approved Striant, a sustained-release buccal testosterone tablet. It is placed in the small depression in the mouth where the gum meets the upper lip, above the front teeth. Once applied, the tablet softens and delivers testosterone through the buccal mucosa, or gums. It is then absorbed directly into the blood stream, bypassing the liver and the rest of the gastrointestinal system. The recommended dosage for Striant is to replace the tablet about every 12 hours, though a different dosing schedule or number of tablets might be required depending on the total testosterone levels of the patient. Some men complain that the tablets fall off a few hours after application.

Some patients find this treatment too cumbersome. Others are concerned about the system shifting out of place or transferring testosterone to sexual partners via the saliva. Others may object to twice-daily dosing and would just as soon use daily gels. A bitter taste and gum inflammation can occur but usually resolves after the first week.

The average wholesale price of a 30-day supply of 30 mg buccal tablets for twice-daily dosing is US$190.30, or approximately US$6.34 a day.

This option has not really caught on, probably for obvious reasons.

PERSONAL COMMENT: I have not tried this option. No particular reason; I guess I was too busy trying other options and the thought of having something stuck to my gums was not really appealing.

Human Chorionic Gonadotropin

Human chorionic gonadotropin (HCG) (not to be confused with human growth hormone, or HGH) is a glycoprotein hormone that mimics LH (luteinizing hormone), produced in pregnancy by the developing embryo soon after conception, and later by part of the placenta. Its role is to prevent the disintegration of the corpus luteum of the ovary and to maintain the progesterone production critical for pregnancy in women. It supports the normal development of an egg in a woman's ovary, and stimulates the release of the egg during ovulation. HCG is used to cause ovulation and to treat infertility in women.

You're probably asking yourself "And I should care because...?" But in men, HCG is also used in young boys when their testicles have not dropped down into the scrotum normally. Additionally, HCG is used to increase testicular size after long-term testosterone or anabolic steroid use (now I've got your attention!).

As mentioned at the beginning of the book, testosterone replacement therapy triggers the hypothalamus to shut down its production of GnRH (gonadotropin releasing hormone). Without GnRH, the pituitary gland stops releasing LH. Without LH the testes (testicles or gonads) shut down their production of testosterone. For males HCG closely resembles LH. If the testicles have shrunken after long-term testosterone use, they will likely begin to enlarge and start their testosterone production shortly after HCG therapy is instituted. HCG jump-starts your testes to produce testosterone and to increase their size.

HCG can be extracted from pregnant women's urine or through genetic modification. The product is available by prescription under the brand names Pregnyl, Follutein, Profasi, and Novarel. Novire is another brand but it is a product of recombinant DNA. Compounding pharmacies can also make HCG by prescription in different vial sizes. Brand names of HCG in regular pharmacies cost around $100 per 10,000 IUs. The same amount of IUs cost around $50 in compounding pharmacies.

What is an IU? When measuring testosterone we spoke in weights of grams and milligrams. HCG is measured not by weight but in IU's, or international units. IU is not about weight but refers to the amount of a substance that produces a particular biologic effect that has been agreed upon as in international standard. The IU from one substance to the next does not mean they have equivalent weights (for example, 1, 000 IU of vitamin C might have a different weight than 1,000 IU of vitamin A). Again, IU is not a weight.

HCG is dispensed as a powder contained in vials of 5, 000 IUs or 10, 000 IUs. These are usually accompanied by another vial of 1 mL (or cc) of bacteriostatic water to reconstitute the powder into a liquid solution. Bacteriostatic water (water with a preservative that is provided with the prescription) is mixed in with the powder to reconstitute, or dissolve, it before injection. This type of water can preserve the solution for up to 6 weeks when refrigerated. Some patients do not use the 1 mL water vials that come with the product and instead get their doctors to prescribe 30 cc bottles on bacteriostatic water so that they can dilute the HCG down to a more workable concentration more practical for those using lower doses of HCG weekly.

HCG is given as an injection under the skin. The number of IUs per injection will depend on how much bacteriostatic water you add to the dry powder vial. If you add 1 mL to a 5,000 IU powder vial, then you will have 5,000 IUs per mL, so 0.1 mL would be 500 IUs. If you add 2 mL to the 5,000 IU dry powder vial, then you will have 2,500 IUs/mL; 0.1 ml (or cc) in an insulin syringe will equal 250 IUs.. If you need to inject 500 IUs, then you inject 0.2 ccs of this mixture. Table 3 provides dilution volumes at different HCG powder/water proportions:

Ultra-fine needle insulin syringes are used to inject HCG under the skin, making this very easy to take even for the needle-phobic. Typical sizes are:

- 1 ml, 12.7 mm long, 30 gauge and
- 0.5 ml, 8 mm, 31 gauge syringes.

Syringes require a separate prescription. Never use the syringe that you used for injecting the bacteriostatic water into the powder for injecting yourself; the needle will be dull (I usually use a regular 23 gauge, 1 inch, 3 ml syringe to load up the water). Remember that you also need alcohol pads to clean the injection area and the tip of the vial. Typical injection sites are the abdominal area close to the navel or in the pubic fat pad. Pinch a little of fat on your abdominals and inject into that pinched area, then massage with an alcohol pad. Discard syringes into the sharps box that can be provided by your pharmacy.

Table 3. HCG Dilution Table

IUs of dry powder HCG	Amount of bacteriostatic water mixed in (cc)	Injection volume for 250 IU (cc)	Injection Volume for 500IU (cc)	Injection volume for 1000 IU (cc)
5,000	5	0.25	0.5	1
5,000	10	0.5	1	2
10,000	5	0.13	0.25	0.5
10,000	10	0.25	0.5	1

Compounded HCG is a lot cheaper than the commercially available pharmaceutical products. Sometimes it is difficult to find commercially available HCG in regular pharmacies.

A review of the literature reveals a wide range of doses of HCG used and that there is very little agreement among physicians. For male infertility, doses ranging from 1250 IU three times weekly to 3000 IU twice weekly (these studies did not include men on testosterone replacement).

Currently there are no HCG guidelines for men who need to be on testosterone replacement therapy and want to maintain normal testicular size and sperm production. A study that used 200 mg per week of testosterone enanthate injections with HCG at doses of 125, 250, or 500IU every other day in healthy younger men showed that the 250 IU dose preserved normal testicular function (no testicular size measurements were taken, however). There are no long-term studies using HCG for more than 2 years.

The best dose of HCG to sustain normal testicular function while keeping estrogen and DHT conversion to a minimum has not been established. Some doctors are recommending using 200–500 IUs twice a week for men who are concerned about testicular size or who want to preserve fertility while on testosterone replacement. Higher doses, such as 1,000–5,000 IUs twice a week, have been used but I believe that these higher doses could cause more estrogen and DHT-related side effects, and possibly desensitize the testicles for HCG in the long term. Some doctors check estradiol levels a month after this protocol is started to determine whether the use of the estrogen receptor modulators tamoxifen (brand name: Nolvadex) or anaztrozole (brand name Arimidex), is needed to counteract any increases in estradiol levels. Estradiol can cause breast enlargement in men (refer to the Gynecomastia section).

A very well known doctor in the field of testosterone replacement, Dr. John Crisler (www.allthingsmale.com), has been using 250-350 IU of HCG on day 5 and 6 after a weekly testosterone injection (two days and one day before the next injection). For men using testosterone gels, the same dose every third day has anecdotally helped to preserve testicular size (the dose of the gel has to be adjusted after a month of HCG to compensate for the increased testosterone caused by HCG). As you can tell, using this product requires a lot of discipline since you have to remember to inject it weekly in addition to your weekly or bi-weekly testosterone injection. But I know of many men who have that type of commitment since they do not want testicular size reduction. And many of us may just be OK with our reduced testicular size as long as testosterone is actually doing its job in improving our sex drive. And some lucky ones do not get testicular atrophy at all on testosterone. So it is a personal decision at the end!

According to Dr. Crisler, using HCG as sole testosterone replacement option does not bring the same subjective benefit on sexual function as pure testosterone delivery systems do—even when similar serum androgen levels are produced from comparable baseline values. However, supplementing the more "traditional" transdermal, or injected options, testosterone with the correct doses of HCG stabilizes blood levels, prevents testicular atrophy, helps rebalance expression of other hormones, and brings reports of greatly increased sense of well-being and libido. But in excess, HCG can cause acne, water retention, moodiness, and gynecomastia (breast enlargement in men).

As you will read in the section "HPGA dysfunction" HCG is also used in a protocol in combination with clomid and tamoxifen to attempt to bring the body's own testosterone production back to normal when someone needs to stop testosterone or anabolic steroids after long-term use.

PERSONAL COMMENT: I have used HCG to reverse testicular shrinkage and it works extremely well. I do have to remind myself that as soon as I stop using it, testicular atrophy will recur. I have recently started using it in small doses (250 IU twice a week) and will report results after a few months on TestosteroneWisdom.com. I get my HCG from compounding pharmacies at $50 per 10,000 IUs.

Clomid (Clomiphene Citrate)

While testosterone replacement is the most commonly used treatment for testosterone deficiency, it can lead to decreased sperm count and possible infertility. It may be a less effective physiologic therapy for patients with secondary hypogonadism due to pituitary dysfunction. Clomiphene citrate (brand name Clomid) is believed by some to allow for restoration of testicular function by restoring physiologic pituitary function in some men with hypogonadism (this statement has not been proven in clinical studies). Clomiphene citrate increases LH and testosterone. It does not appear to downregulate testicular Leydig cell activity, because it blocks testicular estrogen receptors.

Clomiphene citrate is a selective estrogen receptor (ER) modulator approved in 1967 for the treatment of female infertility. It should be noted that most of the data for clomiphene were obtained through studies conducted in women, and good studies with its use in men have yet to be conducted (there is a company setting up research studies to explore the use of clomiphene in men with hypogonadism induced by long term anabolic steroid use). Clomiphene citrate's mechanism of action is primarily as an "antiestrogen." It occupies estrogen receptors and "deceives" the hypothalamus into sensing a low estrogen environment. This activity enhances the hypothalamus' release of GnRH, which impacts the HPGA by stimulating release of FSH and LH from the pituitary. Clomiphene citrate may provide an approach to hormone replacement that is more similar to the normal physiology of the HPGA compared with testosterone replacement therapy, and it may preserve fertility. However, several studies evaluating clomiphene citrate for the treatment of male infertility have produced mixed results. Further study will be needed to clarify the compound's potential utility in this indication.

But can clomiphene improve sexual function in men without the co-current use of testosterone? To answer this question, Dr Guay and his team at the Center for Sexual Function in Peabody, Massachusetts, studied the effect of clomiphene citrate on primary hypogonadism (testicles themselves aren't producing enough testosterone) and erectile dysfunction in 272 men who have never used testosterone. Of these 272 trial participants, 228 completed a four-month regimen of clomiphene citrate dosed at 50 mg three times a week.

Mean age of these 173 men was 54.3 years. After four months of treatment, 75.1 percent of subjects reported improvement in erectile dysfunction including 38.7 percent who reported normal sexual function. The other 24.8 percent reported no change in erectile dysfunction. Serum LH and testosterone levels increased significantly compared with baseline values in all groups (responders, partial responders, and non-responders).

Importantly, clomiphene citrate did not result in supraphysiologic (higher than normal) levels of testosterone in this study, and testosterone levels were maintained within a normal range. Multivariate analysis revealed that age was the patient characteristic most predictive of positive or partial response to clomiphene citrate, with patients aged 55 years and younger more likely to respond compared with patients aged 56 years or older.

For dosing and a protocol that uses clomiphene, HCG and tamoxifen to help to normalize the HPGA after testosterone or anabolic use, please refer to the HPGA dysfunction section and in the Chapter 7 (interview with Dr. Michael Scally).

More studies are needed using clomiphene citrate alone or in combination with HCG and/or tamoxifen or anastrozole so that doctors feel more comfortable prescribing these compounds to help balance the HPGA.

Practical matters to keep in mind: Some men may experience mood changes and feel more emotional when using clomiphene citrate. Clomiphene citrate can be quite expensive, although it can be found at lower prices at compounding pharmacies by prescription. Many doctors do not like to prescribe it due to the limited available data and the fact that it is not approved for men. Some doctors prescribe it off-label and patients pay for it out of their own pockets. It is not a controlled substance under the US Drug Enforcement Agency (DEA).

PERSONAL COMMENT: I have tried using clomiphene as a sole source of testosterone replacement. It did not work. My testosterone remained low and I experienced all symptoms of testosterone deficiency. I have talked to other men who have tried clomiphene with similar lack of efficacy. The discrepancy between my results with Dr Guay's study (which enrolled hypogonadal men with no prior testosterone experience) may be explained by the fact that we had been on testosterone for years before starting clomiphene. No studies have looked into its use in men like me. This is one of the reasons that is simplistic to assume that a drug will work for anyone because studies have shown benefits in some patients. That is the main reason I wanted to try products before writing about them.

Future Products:

Underarm Spray:
In an attempt to reduce the risk of transference of testosterone to others, a company called Acrux is developing Axiron, a testosterone underarm product. Axiron has been studied in 155 men in six countries and 26 sites.

With this product men were permitted to use an underarm deodorant or antiperspirant during the trial. More than half of the men continued to apply an underarm deodorant or antiperspirant as part of their daily routine. An analysis of these subgroups showed that this had no impact on the efficacy of Axiron treatment.

Acrux is targeting to file a New Drug Application (NDA) in the United States for the end of 2009 and Axiron is expected to enter market in early 2011.

Two percent gel:

The same company that is hoping to launch Aveed (Nebido) in the United States, Endo Pharmaceuticals, is expecting to get FDA approval in 2011 for Fortesta(TM) (testosterone) 2% Gel for men diagnosed with low testosterone.

Libigel (from biosantepharma.com):

Results of Phase II

Treatment with LibiGel in BioSante's Phase II clinical trial significantly increased satisfying sexual events in surgically menopausal women suffering from female sexual dysfunction (FSD). The Phase II trial results showed LibiGel significantly increased the number of satisfying sexual events by 238% versus baseline (p<0.0001); this increase also was significant versus placebo (p<0.05). In this study the effective dose of LibiGel produced testosterone blood levels within the normal range for pre-menopausal women and had a safety profile similar to that observed in the placebo group. In addition, no serious adverse events and no discontinuations due to adverse events occurred in any subject receiving LibiGel. The Phase II clinical trial was a double-blind, placebo-controlled trial, conducted in the United States.

Progress and Plans in Phase III

On January 24, 2008, the US FDA notified BioSante that it had completed and reached agreement with BioSante on a Special Protocol Assessment (SPA) for BioSante's Phase III safety and efficacy clinical trials of LibiGel in the treatment of hypoactive sexual desire syndrome (HSDD).

Both Phase III safety and efficacy trials are underway and are double-blind, placebo-controlled trials that will enroll approximately 500 surgically menopausal women each for six-months of treatment.

The last issue beyond efficacy has been the question of safety of testosterone therapy in women, even though there are no data to indicate that low dose testosterone causes any serious adverse events in women. Therefore, in addition to the two Phase III safety and efficacy trials described above, BioSante is conducting one Phase III cardiovascular safety study of LibiGel. The safety study is a randomized, double-blind, placebo-controlled, multi-center, cardiovascular events driven study of between 2,400 and 3,100 women exposed to LibiGel or placebo for 12 months. At the end of 12 months BioSante intends to submit a LibiGel new drug application (NDA) for review and possible approval by FDA. BioSante will continue to follow the women enrolled in the safety study for an additional four years after the NDA submission and possible approval of LibiGel.

BioSante believes it will take approximately 12 months to enroll the women in this multi-national cardiovascular-events-driven safety trial. Therefore, BioSante expects to be able to submit the LibiGel NDA for a potential approval and launch in 2011.

Selective Androgen Receptor Modulators

Oral selective androgen receptor modulators (SARMs) are investigational agents. Studied since 1998, they are still very much in the infancy of their development and marketing. SARMs may be able to provide the benefits of increased muscle mass and bone density, and fat loss that testosterone and other traditional anabolic/androgenic steroids provide but without the unwanted side effects (liver dysfunction or prostatic enlargement). SARMs are not intended to be a form of testosterone replacement therapy. I know, I know – so why am I talking about them? Besides replacement therapy, testosterone and other anabolics can be useful in the treatment of certain aspects of disease. This is a topic close to my heart since this kind of medical use saved my life and that of many others. Excuse me while I digress from the current topic.

Weight loss is common in a number of medical conditions (e.g., HIV/AIDS, burns, trauma, cancer, chronic obstructive pulmonary disease).

The loss of too much weight, especially muscle mass, increases the risk of complications, including death.

Cancer cachexia, or the unintentional loss of muscle mass and body weight, may lead to a loss of protein stores, severe weakness and fatigue, immobility and a loss of independence. It can impair the ability to tolerate and to respond to cancer treatments. An estimated 1.3 million cancer patients in the United States have cancer cachexia. Cancer-induced muscle wasting is thought to be responsible for greater than 20 percent of cancer deaths.

There are no drugs currently approved for the treatment of cancer cachexia.. Physicians often prescribe different medications that have the side of effect of increased appetite in an attempt to fight weight loss. Megace, a progesterone-based appetite stimulant, is commonly used to increase weight. Unfortunately most of this weight consists of fat (lean body mass, not fat gain, has been correlated to increased survival.) Megace also increases the chances for blood clots and bone death.

Anabolics like nandrolone undecanoate and oxandrolone have been prescribed by progressive physicians to treat wasting in patients with non-androgen dependent cancers (colon, throat, lung, stomach, etc.). Androgens are contraindicated for people with prostate and breast cancer, as they can worsen these types of cancers. Anabolics are usually prescribed along with testosterone replacement even if the patient starting them for wasting syndrome has normal testosterone levels. Anabolics have the same inhibiting effect as testosterone on the HPGA and they decrease testosterone blood levels if no testosterone is used in combination with them. Many doctors fail to remember this and treat wasting patients with anabolics alone, which results in loss of sexual function in patients using them for a few weeks. So, testosterone replacement therapy is essential when prescribing oxandrolone or nandrolone to patients with HIV, cancer, or other debilitating wasting conditions.

Oxandrolone (brand name: Oxandrin), an oral anabolic agent, is FDA approved as "adjunctive therapy to promote weight gain after weight loss following extensive surgery, chronic infections, or severe trauma, and in some patients who without definite pathophysiologic reasons fail to gain or to maintain normal weight, to offset the protein catabolism associated with prolonged administration of corticosteroids, and for the relief of bone pain frequently accompanying osteoporosis." (From the product's package insert). Adjunctive means it is an additive or supportive therapy but it does not treat the *underlying* condition directly. In some patients and depending on the dose and duration, oxandrolone can increase liver enzymes and/or decrease high density cholesterol (HDL), the good cholesterol. Both side effects reverse when the drug is stopped. The usual dose for men is 20 mg/day (it can be used in women with wasting at 5-10 mg/day). As previously mentioned, testosterone is needed with it since it reduces testosterone and potentially sexual function after a few weeks in some patients. It is expensive at $1200 per month for 20 mg/day but insurance companies pay for it with some restrictions.

Nandrolone decanoate (brand name: Deca Durabolin), an injectable anabolic steroid, is the most studied anabolic agent for wasting syndrome. It requires a weekly injection of 200-400 mg plus testosterone replacement (100-200 mg testosterone cypionate a week or 5-10 grams of testosterone gel per day). Nandrolone is legally prescribed in an off-label manner to treat wasting syndrome since it is indicated for the management of the anemia of renal insufficiency and has been shown to increase hemoglobin and red cell mass. No liver toxicity has been observed, but decreases in HDL and other side effects typical of testosterone have been observed in those using higher doses. Nandrolone is no longer available in regular pharmacies but it is available cheaply in compounding pharmacies by prescription (there is a list in the Appendix section). The average cost for 200 mg/week is $40 per month and it may produce the same effects on lean body mass than oxandrolone at 20/day. The only drug that is actually approved in the United States for HIV wasting syndrome that does not require an off label prescription is Serostim (human growth hormone made by Serono), although doctors prescribe oxandrolone and nandrolone a lot more due to cost and lower side effects. Depending on the dose used, Serostim can cost $3000 to $6000 per month. This product can cause joint aches, water retention, and diabetes. More details on treatment of wasting syndrome can be found in "Built to Survive" which I co-authored with Michael Mooney (the book is available on Amazon.com in a print or electronic version and has been translated into Spanish).

So back to the SARMs:

Ostarine is an oral agent that has demonstrated the ability to increase lean body mass and improve muscle strength and performance in postmenopausal women, elderly men, and men and women with cancer ca-chexia. Ostarine is made by the company GTx's and has been studied in seven Phase I, Phase II, and Phase IIb clinical trials in 582 subjects.

It had no serious adverse events reported. Ostarine also exhibited no apparent change in measurements of serum prostatic specific antigen (PSA), sebum production (which causes acne), or decreases in blood levels of LH (which hints that it may not affect the HPGA at the doses tested).

SARMs have anecdotally not helped increase sexual function, so they probably will not replace testosterone for treatment of hypogonadism. They also decrease the body's production of testosterone, just like ana-bolic steroids do. So, testosterone replacement will most probably be still required with their use for illness or aging associated loss of lean body mass. We await more data on these interesting compounds as they may have the same clinical benefits as anabolic steroids without the stigma and possibly without their side effects.

-4-

Monitoring Testosterone Replacement Therapy

Testosterone replacement therapy is not without side effects, although most are manageable. I've been taking testosterone replacement for 16 years and for the most part have had few side effects thanks to careful monitoring. It's critical that you are monitored for side effects in addition to your testosterone level. Some men may experience one or more side effects that sometimes go unnoticed until it is too late. In part it is the underground, unmonitored use of testosterone that creates so much bad publicity for a very helpful product.

The first step in the proper monitoring of replacement therapy is providing your doctor with a thorough medical history. Appendix A shows a simple and comprehensive medical history form (courtesy of Dr John Crisler, allthingsmale.com). Patients who would like to be proactive can fill out this form and give a copy to their doctor. It is expected that every doctor have a similar form, although most do not ask questions pertinent to sexual function or on the use of androgens. Let your doctor know about all the medications you take so that medication-induced sexual dysfunction can be ruled out before starting testosterone.

I also strongly believe that if a patient goes to the doctor to obtain a Viagra, Cialis or Levitra prescription, the doctor should check the patient's testosterone blood levels to ensure that it is not the root of the problem. Hypogonadal men may not respond as well to these drugs if their testosterone is not normalized first. Studies combining testosterone and oral sexual enhancement drugs have shown a synergistic effect on sexual benefits. The following suggested guidelines for monitoring testosterone replacement is recommended by several physician groups and practices:

1. You should be evaluated after the first month of therapy to measure your testosterone blood levels. If your doctor doesn't ask, let him know

about your quality of life. Make sure your doctor is aware of your energy level, mood, and sexual function, as well as any potential side effects (tender breasts, urinary flow decrease, moodiness, and acne).

2. When using testosterone, your doctor will want to measure total blood testosterone levels right before the next corresponding injection after the first month (it takes a while for the blood levels to stabilize). If testosterone is >700 ng/dl (24.5 nmol/liter) or <350 ng/dl (12.3 nmol/liter), your doctor will adjust the amount or the frequency of your dose. I mentioned this earlier in the book but it bears repeating here: Some men need to have levels above 500 ng/dl to experience any of the expected sexual function benefits from testosterone. It is important to be honest about when your doctor asks you about your sexual performance.

3. Your doctor will check your hematocrit before starting testosterone, after 3 months and then every year after that. If your hematocrit is above 54%, you may need a therapeutic phlebotomy (read the section "Checking for Increased Blood Thickness (Polycythemia)" for more details.

4. Be ready to have a digital rectal examination done and a prostatic specific antigen (PSA) blood test drawn prior to starting testosterone, and after 3 months. Once every 6 months after that may not be unreasonable, especially in older men. A PSA over 4 ng/ml can be reason for concern and referral to an urologist. Testosterone replacement needs to be stopped if increases in PSA above normal are observed. Note: at the start of testosterone replacement in older men, when testosterone blood levels are rapidly rising, PSA may also increase. This is especially true when testosterone gels are employed, because they elevate DHT more relative to other options. Once testosterone levels have stabilized PSA drops back down to roughly baseline. It is important to allow "steady state" for testosterone fluctuations to stabilize before measuring PSA; a month or so should be sufficient.

5. If you start experiencing breast tenderness, pain or growth, ask your doctor to measure your estradiol blood level using the sensitive assay (not the regular test used for women). Normal range for estradiol in men is 14–54 pg/ml (50–200 pmol/liter). Men who have high estradiol can be prescribed estrogen receptor inhibitors (more details in "Avoiding enlarged breasts (gynecomastia)"

Ensuring Prostate Health—No Link Found Between Androgen Levels and Risk for Prostate Cancer

The prostate is a gland that is part of the male reproductive system. Its function is to store and secrete a slightly alkaline (pH 7.29) a milky fluid which usually constitutes 25-30% of the volume of the semen along with spermatozoa. This alkaline fluid seems to neutralize the acidity in the vagina, prolonging the life span of the sperm. Also, the prostate contains some smooth muscles that help expel semen during ejaculation. It also helps control the flow of urine during ejaculation.

A healthy human prostate is classically said to be slightly larger than a walnut. In actuality, it is approximately the size of a kiwi fruit. It surrounds the urethra just below the urinary bladder and can be felt during a rectal exam.

Prostate cancer

This little gland attracts a great deal of attention in men's health. One of the major issues is related to cancer. Prostate cancer is one of the leading causes of death in men in the United States. As men age, small hidden prostatic lesions become increasingly common. These may or may not become cancerous. These lesions occur in 30 percent of American men over the age of 45, with the prevalence rising to more than 80 percent for men over the age of 80. Genetic factors and life style conditions such as diet are believed to contribute to this transformation.

Doctors use different methods to detect prostate cancer, including prostate-specific antigen (PSA) assays, digital rectal examination (DRE), and transrectal ultrasound. A DRE before starting testosterone replacement therapy and every six months is recommended, especially for men with a family history of prostate cancer or those older than 40 years. Nobody likes having a DRE but your continued good health is worth a few seconds of discomfort. An abnormal rectal exam, a confirmed increase in PSA greater than 2 ng/mL, or PSA of over 4 ng/mL will prompt a health care provider to refer you to a urologist for further evaluation (usually an ultrasound and prostate biopsies).

Admittedly the PSA and the DRE lack sensitivity and specificity. 25 percent of patients with prostate cancer have normal PSA levels (false negatives), while benign prostatic hyperplasia (BPH), a non-cancerous inflammation, may elevate them (false positives). Researchers have found hidden prostatic lesions with needle biopsies in some men with normal PSA level and normal transrectal ultrasound findings. Prostate biopsies are part of routine clinical use of testosterone therapy and are not justified unless a sharp rise in PSA is observed and infections have been ruled out.

Figure 14. The prostate and surrounding organs
(Courtesy of Wikipedia.com)

There has some been confusion regarding testosterone replacement therapy's role in PSA elevation or causing prostate cancer. Prostate cancer is initially androgen-dependent so testosterone therapy should *not* be used by men with prostatic cancer. This does not mean that it causes cancer. A huge pooled analysis of data from 18 studies (consisting of 3,886 men with prostate cancer and 6,438 controls), published in the February 6, 2008 issue of the *Journal of the National Cancer Institute* found that blood levels of androgens and other sex hormones do ***not*** seem to be related to an increased risk for prostate cancer. In short, testosterone therapy does not appear to cause prostate cancer but it can make it worse.

Prostate infection

Another health concern is prostatitis or prostate infection. This is common in aging men and can be a leading cause of an elevated PSA. Your doctor will want to check you for an infection if your PSA unexpectedly increases by checking your urine for white blood cells. If they are high, he may refer you to an urologist who would induce a discharge from your penis to look at it under the microscope. Don't ask me how the urologist does it, ask the urologist!

Benign prostatic hyperplasia

A common health condition is benign prostatic hyperplasia or BPH. It is estimated to occur in 50 percent of men older than 50 years. Increased frequency of urination, frequent trips to the bathroom at night, incomplete voiding, and urgency to urinate indicate possible prostatic inflammation. BPH does not necessarily lead to increased rates of prostate cancer. There have been no prospective, controlled, long-term studies on the effects of testosterone administration on either the development or the progression of BPH. One open label, one-year study that measured prostate size using ultrasound found *no* increase during testosterone replacement therapy, suggesting that the treatment does not cause BPH. Whether testosterone treatment worsens asymptomatic BPH has not been established. Some individuals are more prone to prostatic inflammation when using testosterone.

Another study was conducted by Dr. Michael D. Trifiro at Moores UCSD Cancer Center in San Diego. Dr. Trifiro observed 158 men for 20 years to determine the correlation between serum sex hormones and lower urinary tract symptoms (reduced urinary flow, urgency, and other symptoms associated with BPH). The researchers found no significant associations of total testosterone, estradiol (E2)), testosterone: E2 ratio, DHT, or dehydroepiandrosterone with lower urinary track symptoms or with any measured hormones (published in *BJU International* in December 2009).

Tesosterone replacement therapy is not contraindicated in those with BPH. Men with BPH who need to start testosterone replacement should be observed very closely. The first symptom that worsens with increased BPH is restricted urinary flow and urgency, especially during sleep hours. Many urologists are successfully prescribing medications to ease those symptoms and improve urinary flow in men with BPH. Finasteride (brand name: Proscar), which was approved by the FDA in 1992, inhibits production of dihydrotestosterone (DHT), which is involved with prostate enlargement. Its use can actually shrink the prostate in some men. However, many men using Proscar complain of erectile dysfunction (DHT receptors may be involved in healthy erctions). For men who experience this side effect, other medications may be of help. Proscar has also been found to decrease the risk of prostate cancer in men by 25 percent *over a* seven year period. More studies are ongoing.

The FDA approved the drugs terazosin (brand name: Hytrin) in 1993, doxazosin (Cardura) in 1995, and tamsulosin (Flomax) in 1997 for the treatment of BPH. All three belong to the class of drugs known as alpha blockers. They work by relaxing the smooth muscle of the prostate and bladder neck to improve urine flow and to reduce bladder outlet obstruction.

Terazosin and doxazosin were developed first to treat high blood pressure. Tamsulosin is the first alpha-blocker developed specifically to treat BPH. The main side effects of these drugs are nasal congestion, lowered blood pressure, and rash or itching. Most men using them report fast improvements in their urine flow within one to three days. They end up not having to get up in the middle of the night to urinate, so they sleep better and feel less fatigued during the day.

The most common nonprescription agent used to alleviate symptoms of BPH is the over-the-counter herb saw palmetto (*Serenoa repens*). Extracted from the berry of the saw palmetto shrub, this substance is thought to inhibit 5-alpha reductase (5-·R), thus blocking the conversion of testosterone into DHT, which is responsible for stimulating growth of the prostate gland.

Saw palmetto is generally well tolerated; side effects are infrequent, but include headache and gastrointestinal upset. No known drug interactions are associated with the use of this herb. Some studies found that saw palmetto led to an increase in urine flow rate in men with BPH compared with placebo, with effects comparable to finasteride.

One randomized, double-blind, placebo-controlled study followed men with BPH who took standardized saw palmetto extract 160 mg or placebo twice daily for one year. There was no significant difference found between the saw palmetto and placebo groups in standardized objective urinary symptoms. The incidence of side effects was similar in the two groups. These results cast considerable doubt on the effectiveness of saw palmetto for the treatment of BPH.

Patients who cannot tolerate BPH medications are now using emerging techniques like lasers to vaporize obstructing prostate tissue (www. greenlighthps.com). Talk to your urologist about this if you're interested.

PERSONAL COMMENT: After using testosterone for 17 years, I started to develop a weak urine flow. My doctor gave me prescriptions for several alpha blockers (Uroxatral, Flomax, etc). They worked great but I experienced a rash with each one. My urologist found a prostate infection, which he treated with antibiotics. The infection seemed to linger for months. I then received an ultrasound of my prostate. This test showed that my prostate was not enlarged. Instead it showed that a calcification, caused by a chronic prostatic infection, was blocking my urine flow through my prostate. I got the green light laser procedure done to open up my urethra. It worked great. So, what may seem like BPH may not be! Prostatic infections often go untreated for months since in many cases we may not have symptoms.

Checking for Increased Blood Thickness (Polycythemia)

In addition to increasing muscle and sex drive, testosterone can increase your body's production of red blood cells. This hemopoietic (blood building) effect could be a good thing for those with mild anemia. An excessive production of red blood cells is called polycythemia; it's not a good thing. With polycythemia the blood becomes very viscous or "sticky" making it harder for the heart to pump. High blood pressure, strokes, and heart attacks can occur. This problem is not that common in men taking replacement doses of testosterone but more common in those taking higher bodybuilder doses.

It's important to have your doctor check your blood's hemoglobin and hematocrit.. Hemoglobin is the substance that makes blood red and helps transport oxygen in the blood. Hematocrit reflects the proportion of red cells to total blood volume. The hemoglobin and hematocrit should be checked before starting testosterone replacement therapy, at three to six months and then annually. A hematocrit of over 54 percent should be evaluated. Discontinuation of testosterone may be necessary but there is another option.

Many patients on testosterone replacement who experience polycythemia do not want to stop the therapy due to fears of re-experiencing the depression, fatigue and low sex-drive they had before starting treatment. For those patients, therapeutic phlebotomy may be the answer. Therapeutic phlebotomy is very similar to what happens when donating blood, but this procedure is prescribed by your physician as a way to bring down your blood levels of hematocrit and viscosity.

A phlebotomy of one pint of blood will generally lower hematocrit by about 3 percent. I have seen phlebotomy given weekly for several weeks bring hematocrit from 56 percent to a healthy 46 percent. I know physicians who prescribe phlebotomy once every six weeks because of an unusual response to testosterone replacement therapy. This simple procedure is done in a hospital blood draw facility and can reduce hematocrit, hemoglobin, and blood iron easily and in less than one hour. Unfortunately, therapeutic phlebotomy can be a difficult option to get reimbursed or covered by insurance companies. Your doctor may need to write a letter of medical necessity for it. If you are healthy and without HIV, hepatitis B, C, or other infections, you could also donate blood at a blood bank (a great way to help others!).

The approximate amount of blood volume that needs to be withdrawn to restore normal values can be calculated by the following formula, courtesy of Dr. Michael Scally, an expert on testosterone side effect management. The use of the formula includes the assumption that whole blood is withdrawn. The duration over which the blood volume is withdrawn is affected by whether concurrent fluid replacement occurs.

Volume of Withdrawn Blood (cc)= Weight (kg) × ABV×[Hgb_i - Hgb_f]/[(Hgb_i +Hgb_f)/2]

Where:

ABV = Average Blood Volume (default = 70)

Hgb_i (Hct_i) = Hemoglobin initial

Hgb_f (Hct_f) = Hemoglobin final (desired);

So, for a 70 kg (154 lbs) man (multiply lbs **x** 0.45359237 to get kilogram) with an initial high hemoglobin of 20 mg/mL who needs to have it brought down to a normal hemoglobin of 14 mg/mL, the calculation would be:

CC of blood volume to be withdrawn = 5 x 70 x [20 — 14]/[(20 + 14)/2]
= 75 x 70 x (6/17)
= approximately 1850cc;

One unit of whole blood is around 350 to 450 cc; approximately 4 units of blood need to be withdrawn to decrease this man's hemoglobin from 20 mg/mL to 14 mg/mL.

The frequency of the phlebotomy depends on individual factors, but most men can do one every two to three months to manage their hemoglobin this way. Sometimes red blood cell production normalizes without any specific reason. It is impossible to predict exactly who is more prone to developing polycythemia, but men who use higher doses, men with higher fat percentage, and older men may have a higher incidence.

Some doctors recommend the use of a baby aspirin (81 mg) a day and 2,000 to 4,000 mg a day of omega-3 fatty acids (fish oil capsules) to help lower blood viscosity and prevent heart attacks. These can be an important part of most people's health regimen but they are not a replacement for therapeutic phlebotomy if you have polycythemia and do not want to stop testosterone therapy. It amazes me how many people assume that they are completely free of stroke/heart attack risks by taking aspirin and omega-3 supplements when they have a high hematocrit.

Although some people may have more headaches induced by high blood pressure or get extremely red when they exercise, most do not feel any different when they have polycythemia. This does not make it any less dangerous. If you are using testosterone on your own you need to let your doctor know. Your physician may already suspect some sort of anabolic use if lab results reveal elevated hemoglobin and hematocrit.

PERSONAL COMMENT: I had polycythemia back in the mid-1990s when I was using supraphysiologic doses of testosterone and nandrolone to reverse my HIV-related weight loss. I required two phlebotomies in six months. My hematocrit and hemoglobin eventually normalized without any reason even when using the same doses of testosterone and nandrolone.

Ensuring Liver Health

I mentioned this before but it is well worth repeating. Contrary to what some physicians may think, injectable and transdermal testosterone have **not** been known to cause increased liver enzymes. The same cannot be said for over-the-counter supplements that claim to increase testosterone or growth hormone. Not only do most of them not work, but they could increase your liver enzymes to dangerous levels. This problem has been reported in the past to the FDA. I warn people all the time to be careful about their use. It is always good to check your liver enzymes when blood work is done since it is a cheap test and highly useful in detecting toxicities caused by medications or supplements you may be using.

It is the use of oral testosterone and anabolic formulations (except for oral testosterone undecanoate, commonly used in Canada) that can increase liver enzymes. Many men with hepatitis B or C can be safely treated with replacement doses of testosterone without any liver injury if gels, patches or injections are used. I am very concerned that some of these patients may be denied this important therapy due to potential fears and misconceptions. Some studies have shown an increased incidence of hypogonadism, fatigue, and sexual dysfunction in patients with hepatitis.

Some men like to take supplements to protect the liver against the damaging effects of medications, but very limited data is available on their use. Supplements potentially can interfere with medication blood levels; very little is known about supplement-drug interactions. However, I would like to bring up some supplements with data on liver protection:

- Standardized silymarin (milk thistle herb)—160 mg/three timesday
- Evening primrose oil—1,300 mg/three times/day
- Alpha lipoic acid – 100 – 300 mg/three times/day *Glycyrrhizinate Forte* - Three or more capsules/day, but this may increase blood pressure.
- N-acetyl cysteine – 600 mg/three times/day
- Selenium – 200 mcg twice a day.

I trust the Jarrow and Super Nutrition brands for most of my supplements. Talk to your doctor before starting any supplements!

Monitoring Blood Pressure

High blood pressure or hypertension is another serious medical condition that can go undetected because it often has no symptoms. It's referred to as "the silent killer" for this reason. High blood pressure can cause heart attacks, strokes, headaches, ruin your kidneys, erectile dysfunction and shrink your brain.

Before you start testosterone replacement or an exercise program, it is very important to get your blood pressure under control. This is done through diet, stress management, lowering your salt intake and/or the use of medications. It is a good idea to invest in a home-based blood pressure machine. One usually can be purchased at most pharmacy chains and cost under US$50. Some, like the OMRON HEM-780, can measure blood pressure easily and keep track of changes with time. Take measurements twice a day until you gain control of your blood pressure again.

It is important to have your blood pressure measured during the first month of treatment to ensure that it does not increase with testosterone. The good news is that replacement doses are much less associated with this problem. More serious risks for hypertension are associated with the high testosterone doses associated with performance-enhancing use.

NOTE: Some natural ways to decrease blood pressure are decreasing your salt intake, exercising, keeping a normal body weight for your height, managing stress, and engaging in meditation and yoga. "Erection-friendlier" blood pressure medications like ACE (angiotensin converting enzyme) inhibitors, renin inhibitors, ARB's (angiotensin II receptor blockers), and combinations of them may be required for men who cannot maintain a blood pressure reading under 130/80 mm Hg.

Avoiding Enlarged Breast (Gynecomastia)

Yes, I am talking about breast appearance in men, not women. Gynecomastia is a benign enlargement of the male breast resulting from a growth of the glandular tissue of the breast. It is defined clinically by the presence of a rubbery or firm mass extending concentrically from the nipples. Men who start experiencing this problem complain of pain and tenderness around the nipple area. Gynecomastia is caused by higher than normal blood levels of estradiol, a metabolite of estrogen. As discussed earlier in the book, testosterone can convert into estradiol, DHT, and other metabolites. Men with higher amounts of the enzyme aromatase usually have this problem even at lower doses of testosterone. Growth of this glandular tissue is influenced by a higher fat percentage, older age, excessive alcohol intake, and the use of certain medications. Gynecomastia usually occurs early in testosterone replacement in those who experience this side effect.

In several studies on testosterone replacement, only a very small percentage of people receiving testosterone experience growth of breast tissue. In one HIV-specific study conducted by Dr. Judith Rabkin in New York, she reported that out of 150 men enrolled in the study, two men experienced this adverse reaction. Gynecomastia is much more common among those who use high testosterone doses, such as bodybuilders (they call this "gyno" or "bitch-tits").

How do you manage gynecomastia if it does occur? Lowering the testosterone dose had not proven helpful for the two patients in Dr. Rabkin's study. The use of antiestrogens, such as tamoxifen 10 mg twice daily, with lower doses of testosterone has been effective. Gynecomastia can become permanent if the condition lasts very long although it may reduce in size when the androgen use is discontinued. In the absence of resolution, surgical correction may be necessary in severe cases.

For men who experience enlarged breast size, doctors usually check estradiol levels to determine whether too much testosterone is being converted into estrogen. I do not believe that routine measurement of estrogen is needed for men who have no symptoms of high estrogen (mainly breast tissue enlargement and water retention). For those who have higher than normal estrogen, doctors usually prescribe an antiestrogen medication. One such regimen is anastrozole at 1 mg/day during the first week until nipple soreness and breast enlargement disappear. The dose is then lowered to 0.25 mg a day, or 1 mg twice a week.

A warning: Bringing estrogen down to very low levels could cause health problems in men in the long run. Hair/skin quality and health, brain function, bone density, and other important factors may be greatly influenced by estrogen. However a 12-week study in men using anastrozole at 1 mg a day and 1 mg twice a week found no changes in bone metabolism markers.

The normal production ratio of testosterone to estrogen is approximately 100:1. The normal ratio of testosterone to estrogen in the circulation is approximately 300:1. Estrogen (measured as estradiol) should be kept at 30 picograms per milliliter (pg/mL) or lower. As men grow older or as they gain a lot of fat mass, their estrogen blood levels increase, even to levels higher than that of postmenopausal women.

Medications and Products That Can Cause Gynecomastia

A number of medications have been reported in the medical literature to cause gynecomastia due to decreases in testosterone, increases in estradiol, or both. These include:

- Antiandrogens. These include cyproterone, flutamide, and finasteride. used to treat prostate cancer and some other conditions.
- HIV medications. Sustiva, Atripla, and Videx have been associated with gynecomastia.
- Anti-anxiety medications such as diazepam (Valium).
- Tricyclic antidepressants. These include amitriptyline.
- Glucocorticoid steroids.
- Antibiotics.
- Ulcer medication such as cimetidine (Tagamet).
- Cancer treatment (chemotherapy).
- Heart medications such as digitalis and calcium channel blockers.
- Anabolic steroids
- Substances that have been reported to cause gynecomastia include:
- Alcohol
- Amphetamines
- Marijuana
- Heroin
- Soy and flaxseed- There are conflicting studies but it is something to keep in mind

Exposure to pesticides and byproducts of plastic processing has also been linked to increased estrogen and decreased sperm count in men.

Does Testosterone Suppress the Immune System?

This question is raised out of the confusion over the use of the term "steroid." When somebody is having pain or inflammation and their physician prescribes them a "steroid" or something "steroidal", they are prescribing a corticosteroid (like prednisone) to decrease inflammation. These can have an immunosuppressive effect (sometimes its intended). The "steroid" that you hear about from the media when they are talking about use and abuse by athletes refers to an anabolic steroid (like testosterone). The similarities largely end with their street names.

Some *in vitro* and animal data do suggest that high dose testosterone could be immune suppressive. No such immunosuppressive effect is seen when testosterone was added at replacement concentrations. Several studies using testosterone alone or on combination with oxandrolone or nandrolone in HIV-positive immune compromised patients have found no immune suppressive effect.

Protecting your Heart and Keeping Cholesterol (Lipids) in Check

There is widespread misinformation that testosterone supplementation increases the risk of heart disease. There is no evidence to support this in men younger than 65 years of age. In fact testosterone administration to middle-aged men is actually associated with decreased visceral fat, lower blood sugar concentrations and increased insulin sensitivity. Several studies have shown an inverse relationship between total and free testosterone concentrations and intra-abdominal fat mass, risk of coronary artery disease, and type 2 diabetes mellitus. Testosterone has also been shown to increase coronary blood flow. Similarly, testosterone replacement retards the build-up of plaque in experimental models of atherosclerosis.

In 1994, Phillips and colleagues studied 55 men with angina. They found a strong, positive correlation between very low levels of testosterone and increased severity of coronary artery disease as measured by arteriograms, suggesting that testosterone may actually have a protective effect. This is consistent with the observation that the risk for atherosclerosis increases with age in men, while testosterone levels decrease. Two other smaller studies found that the administration of testosterone decreased risk factors for coronary artery disease.

The European prospective investigation into cancer in Norfolk (EPIC-Norfolk) Prospective Population Study examined the prospective relationship between the body's own (endogenous) testosterone concentrations and mortality due to all causes, cardiovascular disease, and cancer in a nested case-control study based on 11,606 men aged 40 to 79 years surveyed in 1993 to 1997 and followed up to 2003. Among those without prevalent cancer or cardiovascular disease, 825 men who subsequently died were compared with a control group of 1489 men still alive, matched for age and date of baseline visit. Endogenous testosterone concentrations at baseline were inversely related to mortality due to all causes (825 deaths), cardiovascular disease (369 deaths), and cancer (304 deaths). So this study found that in men, endogenous testosterone concentrations are inversely related to mortality due to cardiovascular disease and all causes, and that low testosterone may be a predictive marker for those at high risk of cardiovascular disease.

But there is some emerging contradicting data from a much smaller study that showed that older men who have higher endogenous testosterone (without taking testosterone) may have a higher incidence of heart disease. A large U.S. multicenter study showed that older men with higher testosterone levels are more likely to have a heart attack or other cardiovascular disease in the future. The results were presented at The Endocrine Society's 92nd Annual Meeting in San Diego in June 2010. Study participants were age 65 or older and included 697 community-dwelling men who were participating in the National Institutes of Health-funded study, Osteoporotic Fractures in Men (MrOS). None of these men were receiving testosterone therapy, according to the study abstract.

All subjects had blood tests to determine their testosterone levels. The investigators then divided the men into quartiles, or four groups, of testosterone range to observe trends in rates of coronary heart disease events. This type of heart disease results from plaque-clogged or narrowed coronary arteries, also called atherosclerosis. A coronary heart disease event included a heart attack; unstable angina, which is chest pain usually due to atherosclerosis and which doctors consider a prelude to a heart attack; or an angioplasty or bypass surgery to clear blocked arteries.

During an average follow-up of nearly 4 years, 100 men, or about 14 percent, had a coronary disease event, in particular, heart attacks. After the researchers adjusted for other potential contributing risk factors for heart disease, such as elevated cholesterol, they found that higher total testosterone level relates to an increased risk of coronary disease. Men whose total testosterone was in the highest quartile (greater than or equal to 495 nanograms per deciliter, or ng/dL) had more than twofold the risk of coronary disease compared with men in the lowest quartile (below 308 ng/dL).

In report was published in the New England Journal of Medicine in June 2010 about a study researching the use of testosterone gel in older men that was stopped due to a higher incidence of side effects in men treated with the gel. Participants in this trial that was stopped prematurely, called the Testosterone in Older Men With Mobility Limitations, or TOM, were non-institutionalized men aged 65 and older who had difficulty walking two blocks or climbing 10 steps and whose serum testosterone was 100 to 350 ng/dl. The goal was to recruit 252 men, but only 209 subjects had been enrolled by the time the trial, which started in 2005, was stopped last Dec. 31. Testosterone use had the desired effect of improving the men's muscle strength and mobility. But they also experienced a high rate of adverse effects — not just cardiovascular problems but respiratory and skin problems. Previous studies have shown that In general, older men have more side effects when using testosterone (polycythemia, gynecomastia, high blood pressure, prostatic hyperplasia) and more co morbid conditions. They also require more testosterone to reach normal levels since they have more sex hormone binding globulin that attaches to testosterone and renders it useless. So, physicians should carefully monitor these patients if they decide to provide testosterone replacement. The age cut off when the risk-to-benefit ratio of testosterone changes is not known yet. There are several studies listed in the Appendix that are currently being performed to provide more answers.

So, the jury is still out. But if no complicating factors like high cholesterol, blood pressure or strong family history of heart disease are present, many doctors opt for prescribing testosterone to older men who need it to have a better quality of life.

It is the excessively high doses of testosterone used by athletes and recreational body builders that are linked to significant decreases in the plasma concentration of HDL (high-density lipoprotein - the good cholesterol) and increases in LDL (low-density lipoprotein – the bad cholesterol). Replacement doses of testosterone have been shown to have only a modest or no effect on plasma HDL in placebo-controlled trials. In spite of these studies, some physicians continue to think that testosterone replacement can dramatically increase cholesterol levels.

Given the state of the modern diet, all of us should have our doctor check our cholesterol and triglycerides (another lipid linked with heart disease risk). If you think that you have low testosterone you may already have a problem with your lipids. The recommendations of exercise and diet (low in sugars and animal fats) are for everybody but are especially important for men who have high LDL and high triglycerides at the time of starting testosterone replacement. Testosterone therapy can be an important part of your health regimen but don't start testosterone replacement thinking that it will cure high cholesterol. Sometimes high lipids are related to poor diet, sedentary lifestyle, medication side effects, and/or bad genes. Your treatment for high cholesterol and triglycerides can also include "statin" medications and fibrins prescribed to you by your doctor.

NOTE: I think you're getting why I'm telling you that you need a doctor's supervision when on testosterone. So far you've read about the potential impact on hemoglobin and hematocrit, blood pressure and lipids all of which can negatively affect your cardiovascular health. Imagine the even greater risk of those using testosterone at higher than replacement doses.

Over-the-counter "testosterone boosters" may also cause more problems with lipids. Let your doctor know if you are taking those.

Azoospermia (low sperm count)

Sperm are of course the male reproductive cells found in semen; they are the man's contribution to making a baby. One possible side effect of testosterone replacement is azoospermia or low sperm count. This can mean infertility and is of course an issue if you want to have children.

Adding supraphysiological (above normal) testosterone to the body shuts down sperm production so much that the administration of testosterone injections as a means of male contraception is under study. In study participants azoospermia (low sperm count) usually results within approximately 10 weeks of beginning therapy. Rebound of the sperm count to baseline levels occurs within 6 to 18 months of cessation, and subsequent fertility has been demonstrated.

However, studies have shown that a large proportion of men do not suffer significant decreases in sperm count with replacement doses of testosterone, especially if gels are used. But it is always a good idea for men who want to have children and are on testosterone replacement to consult their urologist. Some of these men may need to discontinue testosterone and wait for their sperm production to normalize if their sperm count is found to be low for impregnating a woman. For men who cannot normalize their sperm count after a few weeks or months of testosterone cessation, a combination of HCG and other gonadotropin hormones may be required.

Some fertility doctors prescribe subcutaneous injections of gonadotropin releasing hormone (GnRH) (brand names: Factrel, Lutepulse) alone. They may also prescribe a combination of HCG at a dose of 1000-2500

IU twice a week plus 75-150 IU of human menopausal gonadotropin (HMG) (brand name: Pergonal or Repodex) three times a week. HMG is a hormone extracted from menopausal women that mimics FSH. Other FSH-like hormones that have been used in place of HMG are human urinary follicle stimulating hormone (Brand name: Fertinex) or recombinant FSH (Brand name: Follistin). As mentioned before, FSH stimulates sperm production in the presence of normal levels of LH and testosterone. These protocols have been able to induce normal sperm production in 5-9 months, so it is important to adhere to it for this long period of time before potential fertility can occur. As you can see, fertility enhancement in men with low sperm counts is a complex issue that needs to be monitored by a qualified fertility physician.

Moodiness

Most people are familiar with the term "roid rage." It is a phenomenon that is occasionally seen among athletes who may be using up to 100 times the medically recommended doses of anabolics and who typically combine several different steroids at once. It usually refers to responses of much greater than expected aggression. For some the term conjures up images of a vein-popping Hulk-like character going on a rampage. Some people unfairly expect this result with any use of testosterone, regardless of the dose used.

In a 1994 study by Drs. **Harrison** Pope and David Katz, published in the *Archives of General Psychiatry* 88 athletes who were steroid users were compared with 68 non-users. Among the men using high doses (defined as more than 1,000 mg anabolic steroids/week), manic as well as hypomanic episodes were reported, in addition to episodes of major depression. In contrast the non-users or athletes using "low" doses (less than 300 mg/week) experienced no manic or depressive episodes. They concluded that psychiatric effects are subtle at physiologic doses but become more prominent at supraphysiologic (above normal) doses.

The testosterone researcher Dr. James Dabbs, studied 692 prison inmates to see whether their natural testosterone levels matched their aggression levels. He wrote, "Aggression is only part of the overall picture relating testosterone to behavior. Connections between testosterone and aggression or other antisocial behavior are very much moderated by social forces." He said that he prefers the term, "rambunctiousness," which suggests in a more neutral manner an increase in overall energy and assertiveness.

In another study by Dr. Judith Rabkin, HIV-positive men with low testosterone were given testosterone supplementation. She observed no major mood effects, but did note increases in self-reported irritability. In fact, this was the side effect most commonly reported in her study: 19 percent (28/150) of the patients noticed that they were uncharacteristically assertive, bossy, "hyper," and/or more prone to anger during the first 12 weeks of treatment. However this was a transient effect for most; only 6 of the 28 reported increased irritability on two consecutive visits. This was seldom a cause for concern to the patient.

Dr C. Wang and colleagues from the University of California-Harbor performed a study to assess the effects of testosterone replacement on changes in mood in 51 hypogonadal men for 60 days. They concluded that testosterone replacement therapy in these men improved their positive mood parameters, such as energy, well/good feelings, and friendliness and decreased negative mood parameters including anger, nervousness, and irritability.

So, it seems that depending on the study that you read, testosterone can improve mood or increase rambunctiousness.

PERSONAL COMMENT: I feel my best when my total testosterone is between 500-1000 ng/dL (mid to upper normal range). My coping mechanisms, outlook, energy level, mental focus, the way I relate to others and productivity are great. Only when I have let testosterone drop is when all of those mood parameters drastically change for the worse (I become more negative in my thinking, more irritable, more fatigued, and don't want to deal with small tasks like calling people back). But we are all different in our response to medicines!

Acne and Baldness

It's an interesting combination isn't it? We usually associate acne with our teen years when our testosterone levels were off the chart and balding as part of getting older. Well, here's the explanation: As I mentioned earlier some testosterone is converted into DHT (dihydrotestosterone). Acne is caused by DHT's stimulating effect on the skin's sebaceous glands; too much oil and sebum are produced and can get infected with bacteria. Hair thinning and balding is caused by DHT's negative effect on the hair follicles.

Patients with mild acne and/or a history of adolescent acne may experience eruptions with testosterone therapy, especially on the back and shoulders.

Dr. Judith Rabkin in New York City studied 150 HIV-positive men who were treated in an open study for 12 weeks with testosterone. Acne was reported by 8 percent (12/150), in one instance leading to study discontinuation.

There are various ways of managing acne.

- Taking a shower right after a workout and using a body scrubbing brush can help remove the excess oil induced by higher DHT.
- Antibacterial soaps (such as Lever 2000) or acne prevention washes and creams with benzoyl peroxide or salicylic acid can also help.
- Getting sun exposure for at least 20 minutes a day seems to benefit some people.
- There are studies that show that taking 50 mg of zinc (plus 3 mg of copper to balance it) can decrease the incidence of acne.
- If the acne is related to an infection, some doctors might prescribe antibiotics (erythromycin topical solution USP, 2 percent, and/or erythromycin 250 mg twice a day is often helpful).
- The use of prescription acne medications like isotretinoin (Accutane) should be done under strict medical supervision since it has been linked to liver problems and mood fluctuations.
- NOTE: Other skin problems in HIV-positive patients, particularly folliculitis, may be confused with acne, but are not related to testosterone levels.

Men who are already losing hair (male pattern baldness or related to a health condition) are most likely to experience hair loss with testosterone therapy. Hair loss was reported by 6 percent of the men during the first 12 weeks of testosterone treatment in one small study,

There are a few options for managing hair loss. Propecia (finasteride, the same drug we previously discussed in the prostate section) is a prescription medication approved for hair loss, more cheaply available as the generic finasteride. Some men have reported erectile problems with this medication since it tends to decrease DHT action. DHT is needed for proper erectile function.

Rogaine® lotion is an over-the-counter product that may be of benefit; it is available at most stores. Nizoral®, an anti-dandruff shampoo available as a prescription and over-the-counter at a lower concentration, may help out too. It wasn't originally intended for this purpose but it seems to help block DHT's effect on hair follicles.

> PERSONAL COMMENT: I really like a product called OC Eight when my face gets too oily (available on amazon.com).

Testicular Shrinkage (Atrophy) and Decreased Ejaculate

Testicular atrophy and decreased ejaculate (amount of semen produced by a man when he climaxes) are common with aging. They also occur in approximately 20 percent of men on long-term testosterone therapy (six months or more).

One helpful treatment for these side effects is the administration of HCG. I've discussed this thoroughly under the section on HCG so I will keep it brief here. HCG stimulates the testicles to retain their size and function while making testosterone. HCG administration is done either as a subcutaneous (under the skin) or intramuscular (into the muscle) injection, both equally effective. A single weekly injection seems sufficient to offset testicular atrophy, although for other conditions HCG is administered several times a week. Many physicians prescribe testosterone injections at a dose of 100 to 200 mg a week with 500 to 1000 IU of HCG weekly.

Some urologists have asked patients to estimate their previous testicular size using an orchidometer (Genentech Inc.), and then measured testicular change with HCG treatment. A return to original size has occurred.

Hypothalamic-Pituitary-Gonadal Axis (HPGA) Dysfunction

If you do a quick review of Figure 1 back in chapter 2 and of the sections on HCG and Clomid in chapter 3 you will remember that low testosterone is caused by a problem somewhere in the HPG axis(also called HPT axis).

I am adding Figure 1 here again for the purpose of explaining one of the most important and neglected side effects of using testosterone or anabolic steroids.

The HPT Axis

What you also need to know is that testosterone replacement therapy itself can lead to further HPGA dysfunction. Supplemental testosterone can inhibit the release of the body's own testosterone production through negative feedback inhibition on LH levels. This feedback inhibition also results in suppression of FSH levels, leading to suppression of sperm production (spermatogenesis).

Some men need to stop using testosterone or other androgens because side effects are a problem (e.g. low sperm count interferes with their goal to have children). Most physicians advise the patient to just stop testosterone without thinking about the possible consequences of the hypogonadal state after treatment cessation. Will the patient be worse off than when he started?

Not all studies show a shutdown of the HPGA in patients after testosterone cessation. In a study previously mentioned in the Moodiness section, Dr. Rabkin compiled data for 42 patients who were treated with testosterone for 12 weeks and then randomized (double blind) to receive placebo injections for six weeks. At week 13 (one week after their first placebo injection and three weeks since the last active injection), mean testosterone level was 286 ng/dL. At week 15 (after 2 placebo injections), mean testosterone level was 301, and after week 17 (after 3 placebo injections), mean serum level was 324 ng/dL. None of these values was statistically different from the mean baseline testosterone level of 308 ng/dL. These data suggest that for men who were already hypogonadal there was no further decline in the body's production of testosterone once testosterone therapy was discontinued after 12 weeks of use. It is not known if longer term testosterone use would have the same results.

When high-dose testosterone use (as in bodybuilding) is discontinued the HPGA dysfunction that occurs when it is stopped may be a lot more pronounced. Stopping treatment may cause the patient to suffer all the symptoms of hypogonadism for weeks or months. In some cases a specific medical protocol is required for HPGA normalization.

There is no controlled data from studies using any protocols to accelerate the normalization of normal testosterone production in men who have used either supplemented physiologic (normal) or supraphysiologic (above normal) doses of testosterone for long periods.

For men who had normal testosterone before starting testosterone or anabolic steroids (athletes, bodybuilders or people with wasting syndrome) and who want or need to stop those compounds, some physicians have attempted to jump-start testicular testosterone production using a combination of products that have different effects on the HPGA and estrogen receptors. One such physician is Dr. Michael Scally from Houston (read the interview in Chapter 7) who presented a poster at the Lipodystrophy and Adverse Reactions in HIV conference in San Diego in 2002 that reported the use of a protocol to normalize testosterone production in HIV-positive patients after prolonged anabolic steroid and testosterone use for their wasting syndrome.

The protocol consisted of the use of HCG, clomiphene citrate, and tamoxifen (read about each of these products in their respective sections). Treatment takes place over two discrete intervals. The first treatment interval is to initiate the restoration of gonadal function. The second interval is to restore the hormonal pathways among the hypothalamus, the pituitary and the gonads. The medications are initiated simultaneously after cessation of androgens when it is expected that the body would try to start to slowly make its own testosterone. If the kind of testosterone that the patient used is known (the most common one in the United States is depo testosterone or testosterone cypionate), its half-life in the body can be estimated so that the date to begin the medical protocol can be predicted with some accuracy to assess a time when no pharmaceutical testosterone remains in the body.

The protocol for HPTA normalization contains:
First 15 days:
HCG 2,500 IU (subcutaneous) once every other day;
Clomiphene citrate 50 mg orally twice a day; and
Tamoxifen 20 mg orally once a day.

A satisfactory testosterone level on day 15, typically 350 ng/mL or greater, is followed by the oral medications (no HCG) for an additional 15 days. This protocol has not been tested in many patients but has shown good results in restoring HPGA in a month. I know that this sounds like a long time but without treatment the body's restoration process would take about the same length of time that somebody was using androgens. In some, HPGA function and testosterone production never returns to normal. Hopefully we will see data on approaches like this one used in patients who need to stop testosterone or anabolics after long term use.

Erectile Function and Fatigue- What Happens When Testosterone Replacement Fails to Improve Them?

Most men find that their sexual desire increases after they start testosterone replacement. Sexual dreams and nighttime/morning erections may be more easily achievable, but in some cases testosterone alone does not make erections strong or lasting enough for successful intercourse.

For these men the use of prescription phosphodiesterase type 5 inhibitor (PD-5) medications like *Viagra, Cialis, and Levitra*—may be needed in combination with testosterone replacement. However, some men do not respond well to these oral agents or have side effects such as headaches, nasal congestion, flushing, gut problems, and, in the case of Cialis, back pain. Cialis may last longer than the others (36 hours compared to 4 hours for Viagra or Levitra), but so may its side effects. Some men take Claritin and ibuprofen with these drugs to pre-treat nasal congestion and headaches, respectively. Cialis is also approved for daily use at 5 or 10 mg/ day dose (regular dose is 20 mg/day). They are available by prescription but I have heard that some men are ordering them without a prescription from overseas websites to save money (overseas sources can be ten times cheaper than products in the United States). This book does not endorse the use of these drugs without a prescription, but it is my duty to mention facts about what is happening out in the real world.

Note: If erectile dysfunction is not improved while on testosterone, ask your doctor about adjusting your dose of testosterone. Ensure that your total testosterone level is between 500 and 1000ng/dL. Also, have your doctor check your blood levels of estradiol; if too much testosterone is converted into this female hormone as it may cause sexual dysfunction (.can be treated with low dose Arimidex). Low levels of thyroid hormone, infections, lack of sleep, alcohol, smoking, medications and depression also can cause erectile dysfunction in the presence of normal testosterone levels. Last but not least, lack of attraction for our sexual partner can get in the way of achieving a strong erection.

Other options for men who need an extra erectile boost while using testosterone replacement:

Yohimbine—Available over-the-counter or by prescription (Yocon); increases sex organ sensitivity. It can raise blood pressure and cause insomnia and anxiety, so talk to your doctor. A small study showed that men who used yohimbine with the amino acid arginine had better erections (read section on supplements in this book)

Muse (alprostadil)—this is a prescription pellet that inserts into the penis to produce an erection. Not very popular.

Trimix or Quadmix—Available by prescription from compounding pharmacies. These are mixtures of prostaglandins and papaverine that increase blood flow and retention into the penis. Prostaglandins are mediators and have a variety of strong physiological effects, such as regulating the contraction and relaxation of smooth muscle tissue. Prostaglandins are not hormones and they are not produced at one discrete site, but rather in many places throughout the human body.

Trimix is a mixture of two prostaglandins (phentolamine and alprostadil) plus papaverine (a vasodilator medication) that increase blood flow to the penis and cause strong and lasting erections, with or without sexual stimulation. These compounds appear to act together to increase arterial inflow, dilate smooth muscles, and restrict venous outflow promoting erectile rigidity with greater success and in smaller doses than if these compounds were used as single therapies.

An example of a dosage combination for tri-mix is 10 micrograms of alprostadil, 500 micrograms of phentolamine and 15 mg of papaverine. Dosing of tri-mix preparations has not been standardized.

Trimix is injected directly into the side of the penis through a fine-gauge "insulin-style" needle in very small amounts (0.1-0.33 cc) that increase blood flow to the penis. It results in strong and lasting erections. The main potential side effect are hematomas (bruising), fibrosis if used too frequently and on the same injection site, pain, and dangerously long-lasting erections (priaprism). Priaprism may sound great but this can literally kill your penis by causing gangrene of the tissue after stagnant blood coagulates inside it. I know men who had to go to an emergency rooms 8 hours after having used too much Trimix and have the blood drained from their penis. To ensure perfect injection technique and dosing, it is imperative to be trained on how to dose this with the help of an urologist.

Compounding pharmacies sell two types of Trimix formulations: Freeze dried (powder to be mixed later with water) or pre-mixed vials. Some men find the freeze dried form not to be as effective.

It is extremely important to remember never to use Viagra, Cialis, or Levitra before or at the same time as you use Trimix. This is a dangerous combination that can increase the risk of priaprism. Be particularly careful with Cialis since it can stay in your blood stream for a longer time. I know someone who had priaprism since he had forgotten he had taken Cialis two days before using Trimix.

Most men who use Trimix love it, even if they have had to learn the hard way about priaprism during one instance. Most of these men did not respond well or had too many side effects to oral agents like Viagra or Cialis.

For instructions on how to inject Trimix, read:

www.infertility-male.com/erectdys/injxn1.htm

For instructions for physicians on how to treat priaprism in the unfortunate case that it happens:

emedicine.medscape.com/article/777603-diagnosis

A 10 cc bottle of Trimix can cost from $70 to $100 in compounding pharmacies. If 0.15 ccs are needed per erection, this bottle can be good for 67 erections. In comparison with Cialis and Viagra ($16 a pill), this option seems economical.

Caverject— This is an injectable form of alprostadil. Injections of alprostadil have been reported to cause pain, bleeding, hematomas and scar tissue leading to Peyronie's Disease (excessive curvature of the penis) in some patients. Caverjet is available by prescription and it is not a compounded product, so some doctors who are not comfortable prescribing compounded products feel more at ease prescribing it. However, it is not as effective as Trimix, it requiresa large injection volume, and it comes preloaded in syringes with thick needles. It is also 10 times more expensive than Trimix but several insurance companies pay for it (Trimix is rarely covered by insurance). This injection into the penis that produces an erection that can last 1 to 2 hours. It has a larger injection volume than Trimix and is a lot more expensive, unless your insurance pays for it. Follow instructions from your urologist since overdosing can also cause priaprism.

*Penile restriction rings—*These rubber or leather restricting bands (commonly known as "cock rings") can be very effective at maintaining erections after the penis fills up with blood. Be careful not to use it too tight. Neoprene and leather rings are the most common. They can be found online.

Other options are penile vacuum devices and penile implants. Due to the scope of this book, these two options will not be reviewed. Plenty of information can be found by Googling those terms.

Medications that could cause decreased sex drive or erectile dysfunction:

Medications can cause erectile dysfunction in some men. A great review of all studies of drugs that affect sexual function in men was provided by Dr Walter K.H. Krause in his book "Drugs Compromising Male Sexual Health". He was able to identify evidence from different studies (many uncontrolled and small) about the common classes of prescription medications that can cause erectile dysfunction. It is not known if testosterone replacement can counteract the effects of these medication classes. Among the medications are:

- Antidepressants: Selective serotonin reuptake inhibitors (SSRIs), tricyclic antidepressants, monoamine oxidase inhibitors
- Blood pressure medications (antihypertensives): Alpha andregenergic antagonists, beta-blockers, diuretics, guanethidine, methyldopa
- Narcotics and opiates
- Barbiturates and benzodiazepines
- Hormone related products: Anabolic steroids, antiandrogens used in prostate cancer, estrogens, medroxyprogesterone, 5-alpha-reductase inhibitors
- Anti-acids: Histamine 2 receptor antagonists, proton pump inhibitors
- Cholesterol –lowering agents: Bile acid sequestrants, fenofibrates, statins

Fatigue
If no improvements in fatigue are observed after 6 weeks of testosterone replacement, factors beyond hypogonadism may be present.

Thyroid and adrenal function should be checked to ensure that those two glands are working properly Sleep apnea can also be a factor involved in the failure to improve stamina. Depression may still need to be addressed with the proper medications and counseling.

Thyroid Function:
The thyroid is a butterfly-shaped endocrine gland located in the lower front of the neck. It produces thyroxine or T4, which is converted to tririodothyronine, or T3. T4 production is controlled by thyroid stimulating hormone or TSH, a hormone produced by the pituitary. Hypothyroidism, or low thyroid hormone, can cause sexual dysfunction as well as depression, fatigue, dry skin and hair, weight gain and increased sensitivity to the cold. Blood tests to measure TSH, T4 and T3 are readily available and widely used.

The American Thyroid Association (thyroid.org) has great comprehensive information on how to determine if you have hypothyrodism that could be causing your fatigue.

Adrenal Function:
The adrenal glands, located in the abdomen above the kidneys, regulate stress in the human body. When the body encounters an emergency situa-

tion, the adrenal glands release hormones, such as adrenaline, that enable the body to respond accordingly. You may have encountered this reaction, called the "fight or flight" response, if you have encountered danger, fear or shock. Adrenal fatigue is the controversial idea that the adrenal glands can become worn out, creating illness, if continually over stimulated. Proponents of the "adrenal fatigue" theory hold that the adrenal glands may be over worked in some individuals and therefore become "fatigued" and unable to produce sufficient hormones. When your adrenal glands become exhausted, your natural cortisol levels drop significantly. Cortisol is your naturally occurring stress hormone. In addition to low sex drive and infertility, symptoms of adrenal fatigue may include chronic fatigue, low blood pressure and low blood sugar, dizziness, headaches, anxiety or panic attacks, depression,and other equally debilitating reactions.

Some doctors may prescribe low doses of corticoid steroids if your morning levels of cortisol (measure by blood, saliva or urine tests) are low. But be careful with corticoid steroids since they can increase fat mass and decrease bone density if given in doses that exceed what the healthy adrenals would produce.

DHEA:

The adrenal glands also produce dihydroepiandrosterone (DHEA), the most abundant hormone found in the blood stream. The body uses DHEA as the starting material for producing the sex hormones testosterone and estrogen in men. Studies have shown that it only increases testosterone in women. The production of DHEA diminishes in most people after age 40. In people aged 70 years, DHEA levels will be approximately 30 percent lower than what they were at age 25. Low blood levels of DHEA have been associated with many degenerative conditions.

Some controversial and non-conclusive studies have shown that people with immune deficiencies and fatigue may benefit from supplementation with this hormone. It is still available over-the-counter in the United States. This may change soon due to a new bill passed by Congress that classifies it as a performance-enhancing steroid (no studies have shown that it has such effect).

One study showed that women with the correct levels of DHEA can convert it into testosterone as their body needs while men do not benefit to the same degree. You need a blood test to know if you have low DHEA-S since most of the DHEA converts into this sulfated form. Common doses for women are 5to 30 mg a day, while men tend to benefit from 25-100 mg per day (to bring low levels of DHEA-S to normal)

All the hormones mentioned can be tested with blood tests or by using the easy-do-it-at-home mail order saliva hormone tests that are permissible without a prescription. Mail-order saliva tests for testosterone, DHEA-S, estradiol, and cortisol are offered by Great Smokies Laboratory at 1-800-522-4762.

NOTE: Do not use DHEA supplements unless your blood levels of DHEA-S are low. If low, start at a low dose and get your DHEA-S tested again after a month. Men who use DHEA supplements may have problems with higher estrogen levels since this hormone can also metabolize into estradiol. This could result in gynecomastia and water retention. If you start taking DHEA, have your blood levels checked to make sure they are not above normal. There are many claims about DHEA being an anti-aging and an anti-cancer cure, but *none* of these claims has been substantiated with strong data.

Sleep Apnea:

Sleep apnea is a sleep disorder in which the patient briefly stops breathing or breathes shallowly many times during sleep and therefore does not get enough restful sleep; oxygen levels drop in the blood, starving the brain of oxygen. In addition to causing daytime fatigue, it can increase blood pressure and cardiovascular risks. Testosterone-replacement therapy has been associated with exacerbation of sleep apnea or with the development of sleep apnea, generally in men who use higher doses of testosterone or who have other identifiable risk factors for sleep apnea (high body weight, thick necks, snoring, alcohol consumption, and others). Upper-airway narrowing does not seem to be caused by testosterone replacement therapy, suggesting that testosterone replacement contributes to sleep-disordered breathing by central mechanisms rather than by means of anatomical changes in the airway.

If your spouse or partner complains that you snore loudly at night and you suffer from fatigue, tell your doctor. The only real way to find out if you have sleep apnea is to have your doctor refer you to a sleep lab for a sleep study. If you are diagnosed with sleep apnea, a Continuous Pressure Airway Pressure (CPAP) machine can be prescribed to help you open up your airways with a small air pump while you sleep. Some people love it while some hate wearing a mask while being hooked up to a machine at night. I have seen men regain their quality of life after starting CPAP. It is paid by insurance, Medicare and most HMOs.

Stimulants:

Some physicians prescribe drugs like Nuvigil, Ritalin or Adderall when everything else fails.

Armodafinil (brand name Nuvigil) is used to treat excessive sleepiness caused by narcolepsy (a condition of excessive daytime sleepiness) or shift work sleep disorder (sleepiness during scheduled waking hours and difficulty falling asleep or staying asleep during scheduled sleeping hours in people who work at night or on rotating shifts). Armodafinil is also used along with breathing devices or other treatments to prevent excessive sleepiness caused by obstructive sleep apnea/hypopnea syndrome. Armodafinil is in a class of medications called wakefulness-promoting agents. It works by changing the amounts of certain natural substances in the area of the brain that controls sleep and wakefulness. Some insurance companies do not want to pay for it. It is not an amphetamine and it does not require a special prescription since it not a class III DEA regulated drug. Many doctors have samples so that you can try it before you commit to using it.

Ritalin and Adderall (both come in cheaper generics) are also being prescribed to people with severe fatigue that does not respond to usual means.

Methylphenidate (brand name Ritalin) is used as part of a treatment program to control symptoms of attention deficit hyperactivity disorder (ADHD) in adults and children. Methylphenidate (Ritalin, Ritalin SR, Methylin, Methylin ER) is also used to treat narcolepsy. Methylphenidate is in a class of medications called central nervous system (CNS) stimulants. It works by changing the amounts of certain natural substances in the brain

Adderall is a brand-name psychostimulant medication composed of racemic amphetamine aspartate monohydrate, racemic amphetamine sulfate, dextroamphetamine saccharide and dextroamphetamine sulfate, which is thought to work by increasing the amount of dopamine and norepinephrine in the brain. Adderall is widely reported to increase alertness, libido, concentration and overall cognitive performance while decreasing user fatigue. It is available in two formulations: IR (**I**nstant **R**elease) and XR (e**X**tended **R**elease). The immediate release formulation is indicated for use in Attention Deficit Hyperactivity Disorder (ADHD) and narcolepsy, while the XR formulation is approved for use only with ADHD. In the United States, Adderall is a Schedule II drug under the Controlled Substance Act due to having significant abuse and addiction potential. It requires a triplicate prescription in many states.

If you and your doctor decide that stimulants are a reasonable option, you will need to review the many potential drug interactions, physical health and mental health complications that can occur.

Over-the-Counter Supplement: SAMe

SAMe (SAM-e, S-adenosyl-methionine, or S-adenosyl-L-methionine) is a naturally occurring compound that is found in every cell in the body It is produced within the body from the essential sulfur-containing amino acid methionine. Protein-rich foods are sources of this amino acid.

SAMe is generally considered safe when taken in appropriate doses. People with bipolar (manic/depressive) disorder should be aware that it could trigger a manic phase. People taking standard antidepressants, including MAO inhibitors, SSRIs, and tricyclics should not take SAMe except on a physician's advice. It is fairly well tolerated but be it can cause jitteriness or gut problems in some. Taking SAMe with meals can reduce these adverse effects.

I am convinced this supplement works for depression and fatigue. I have taken 400 mg twice a day for a few months and can definitely feel a difference. I actually get reminded when I do not take it by my having decreased energy. An added bonus is that it can also decrease liver enzymes.

SAMe is not cheap. There are many different manufacturers but I use the Jarrow Formulas brand, as I trust their quality control. It comes in foil-protected 200 mg-capsules since it tends to lose its effectiveness when exposed to air.

Here is a summary of studies that show that it works as well as commonly prescribed antidepressants, and also some data on liver function and arthritis pain:

www.healthyplace.com/Communities/Depression/treatment/alternative/sam-e.asp

I am also including a study done at ACRIA that also found benefits in treating depression in those living with HIV:

www.pubmedcentral.nih.gov/articlerender.fcgi?artid=535560

Talk to your doctor before taking this supplement. Do not stop taking your antidepressants to switch to SAMe since it has not been fully studied in large controlled studies.

PERSONAL COMMENTS: Because of terrible bouts with fatigue in the past, I was referred to a sleep lab and diagnosed with mild sleep apnea. I tried CPAP with different masks (they are smaller ones with "nose pillows" and many other designs, so don't give up early without trying different styles). I could not get used to it. I have had my thyroid and adrenal functions checked without finding any problems. I have tried Nuvigil, Adderall, and SAMe with good results for my fatigue. Unfortunately I get anxious if I use them for long periods, so I only use them as needed. What has made the most difference, besides keeping my testosterone in the upper side of the normal range, is going to bed around the same time at night and waking up also at the same time. Traveling and other factors can interfere with maintaining a normal sleep cycle, but the fact is I need to listen to my body's needs. I can usually be tired enough to get better sleep by the time bedtime arrives if I avoid caffeine after 3 pm and don't exercise too late at night,

-5-

Supplements

Supplements That Claim to Improve Sexual Function and/or Testosterone

Many people either don't trust big drug companies or they prefer the idea of using something they see as "natural" or "herbal". Therefore I'm going to address a few of these. Please keep in mind a general rule about supplements: They are not regulated by the FDA. This leads to a wide range in potency of the product between manufacturers (one reason it can make some studies hard to verify). I have always turned to the people at the non-profit organization Houston Buyers Club (houstonbuyersclub. com) for assistance in choosing my supplements.

Korean red ginseng

Two double-blind, placebo-controlled trials, involving a total of about 135 people found evidence that Korean red ginseng may improve erectile function when compared with placebo. A dose of 900 mg was given three times daily and the study period was 8 weeks.

In an analysis combining the results of six controlled trials, researchers found some evidence supporting the benefits of Korean red ginseng. There are doubts about this conclusion as these studies were small size and non-validated.

L-arginine

L-arginine is an amino acid with many functions in the body. One of these is its role in the production of nitric oxide which helps relax blood vessels.

This relaxation is essential in the development of an erection. Drugs like Viagra increase the body's sensitivity to the natural rise in nitric oxide that occurs when we get sexually excited.   Another approach might be to to raise nitric oxide levels, which led to the idea of trying L-arginine.

Oral arginine supplements may increase nitric oxide levels in the penis and elsewhere. The main data that generated some interest in the use of arginine for erectile dysfunction came from a small double-blind trial in which 50 men with erectile dysfunction received either 5 g of L-arginine or placebo daily for six weeks (**NOTE**: a capsule contains 500 mg, so 10 capsules a day!). More men in the treated group experienced improvement in sexual performance than in the placebo group. A double-blind crossover study of 32 men found no benefit with 1,500 mg of arginine given daily for 17 days. The signficant difference in dose and shorter course of treatment may explain the discrepancy between these two trials.

L-arginine has been advertised as "natural Viagra" but there is little evidence that it works. Drugs based on raising nitric oxide levels in the penis have not worked out for pharmaceutical developers; the body seems to adjust to the higher levels and maintain the same level of response.

NOTE: Large doses of L-arginine can activate the herpes virus in those who have been exposed to it. You may want to take medication for herpes treatment if you decide to use this supplement. L-arginine is also commonly used in bodybuilding supplements since it can cause transient increases in growth hormone.

Yohimbine and yohimbe

Yohimbine HCl is an indole alkaloid found in the bark of the *Pausinystalia yohimbe* tree. Yohimbe bark has been used in Africa for centuries as an aphrodisiac. It is available as a supplement but is also available by prescription in the United States under the trade-name Yocon. It too helps with erections by relaxing blood vessels in the penis.

Yohimbine has been studied in combination with L-arginine. One study of 45 men found that one-time use of this combination therapy an hour or two before intercourse improved erectile function in those with only moderate erectile dysfunction. Arginine and yohimbine were both taken at a dose of 6 g, which would require a lot of capsules (if taken in powder form a tea spoon has 5 g). All the related studies were very small.

I doubt that there are future larger studies planned since we now have effective erectile dysfunction drugs that work.

NOTE: Yohimbine (and yohimbe) present a number of safety risks related to increased heart rate, blood pressure, insomnia, anxiety, and liver/kidney dysfunction. It is best to use this under physician supervision.

PERSONAL COMMENT: I have taken Yocon and found it too "speedy" for me.

Carnitine

Carnitine is a compound that helps transport fatty acids for the generation of metabolic energy. In addition to its apparent benefit for diabetes, the heart and affecting bone mass it may have benefit with erectile dysfunction. Propionyl-l-carnitine at 2 g/day plus acetyl-l-carnitine also at 2 g/day and testosterone (testosterone undecanoate 160 mg/week) were separately compared with placebo. The results indicated that both carnitine and testosterone improved erectile function; however, while testosterone significantly increased prostate volume, carnitine did not. Other studies seem to indicate that propionyl-l-carnitine at 2 g/day enhanced the effectiveness of sildenafil (Viagra) in a small group of men with diabetes who were not responding to sildenafil on at least eight occasions.

PERSONAL COMMENT: I have taken these two forms of carnitine and can honestly say that I have not felt any difference in the erectile department.

Zinc

Zinc is an essential mineral important for many aspects of health. Severe zinc deficiency is known to negatively affect sexual function. Since marginal zinc deficiency is relatively common, it is logical to suppose that supplementation with zinc may be helpful for some men. This hypothesis has only been studied in men receiving kidney dialysis but the results were promising. You can take too much zinc, so check with your doctor about how much is enough.

Maca and other herbal products

The herb maca (Lepidium meyenii) is another supplement advertised as "herbal Viagra" (it is an attention-getter, isn't it?). In one study of rats, maca enhanced male sexual function. For those of you who aren't rats, there is one published human trial. In this small, 12-week, double-blind, placebo-controlled study, use of maca at 1,500 mg or 3,000 mg increased male sexual desire but no data was shown on the quality of erections. The claims that it increases testosterone are not true.

There are other herbs that have been promoted as improving sexual function in men. Among these are Ashwagandha, Avena sativa (oat straw), eleutherococcus (the so-called Siberian ginseng), L-citrulline, *Macuna pruriens*, molybdenum, muira puama or potency wood (you have to love the name), pygeum, *Polypodium vulgare*, Rhodi-ola rosea, saw palmetto, schisandra, suma, traditional Chinese herbal medicine, deer or antelope velvet antler, and Tribulus terrestris.   There are no well-designed, controlled scientific studies that support any of those claims.

Many herbal supplements that claim to improve sexual function have been found to contain Viagra or Cialis purchased in China at cheaper prices. The FDA has stopped those companies from selling them but many keep reappearing in the unregulated supplement market.

All supplements that actually increase testosterone, such as androstenedione, are considered performance-enhancing drugs.   They have been banned in the United States. This is just as well as they only increased testosterone for a few hours and had the potential to cause liver problems. New supplements keep appearing on the market and claim to increase the body's production of testosterone or growth hormone. Be very skeptical about those claims and do not waste your money on them!

The best and safest way to supplement your testosterone is to *use approved products under your physician's supervision and care.*

-6-

Miscellaneous Health Tips to Support Healthy Testosterone

I guess this is the "good news, bad news" part of my book. Yes, testosterone therapy can be of tremendous benefit in restoring your energy and sense of well-being. No, you shouldn't rely on hormone replacement as being the only change that you make in your health regimen. Better health involves some important lifestyle choices. You've probably heard some of these from your doctor, family or anybody who really cares about you. I've also included other tips based on my own experiences.

Tips for Maximizing Your Health and Response to Testosterone Replacement Therapy

- Exercise with weights/machines three to four times a week for no more than one hour; this helps build muscle. On alternate days do cardiovascular exercise (elliptical trainer, fast walking, light jogging, etc.) for at least 30 minutes a day; this helps with stamina and overall health. Make sure that you sweat! Discuss your exercise program with your doctor before you start.
- At the start of any exercise program and every three months measure your chest, thighs, arms, and abdomen. Weigh yourself weekly.
- It is not a bad idea if you are over 40 to ask your doctor for a full body DEXA (dual X Ray Absorptiometry) scan so that you can know how many grams of muscle, fat and bone you have in every part of your body, and then repeat every three years to monitor changes. Sometimes it is difficult to find a radiology clinic that does full body DEXAs since

they are usually accustomed to doing only DEXA's of the hips or spine area for post menopausal women with bone loss.
- Take at least a multivitamin a day with meals. I like the Energy Pack from Super Nutrition.
- Motivate yourself with a buddy or support system. I don't mean just for exercise either; surround yourself with some wise and up-beat people.
- If you have to use stimulants, such as coffee and green tea, use them only in moderation.
- Get good quality sleep. Talk with your doctor if you're not getting it.
- Manage stress with relaxation techniques and hobbies. Learn to let go of anger and unrealistic expectations.
- Get at least 20 minutes a day of sunshine (avoid the face, though). Your body needs it to make vitamin D for bone health. Get your vitamin D blood levels checked and supplement at with at least 2000 IU per day if found to have low blood levels (ask your doctor about this test).
- Sweat. Use a pedometer to try to walk at least 10,000 steps a day. Increase your cardio by parking far, taking the stairs, walking the dog, or dancing. Make it fun!
- Choose your supplements wisely. Beware of companies claiming that their "growth hormone precursors" work; they don't. Most weight loss supplements have stimulants that can affect mood and increase blood pressure and cardiovascular risks.
- Treat depression quickly with exercise, therapy, antidepressants, and a good support system
- Get a Pneumovax vaccine every five years. Pneumovax is a vaccine against bacterial pneumonia.
- If you've never had hepatitis A or B, ask your doctor about getting vaccinated against them.

How to Protect Your Heart

- Do not smoke!
- Manage stress and keep your blood pressure in check.
- Decrease high triglycerides with Omega 3 fatty acids (cold water fish oils) and by cutting down on sugars. The American Heart Association (AHA) recommends at least two 3 oz servings of fish per week. Some experts recommend eating four 3-ounce servings of fatty fish per week

for people with heart disease or cardiac risk factors. The following have higher levels of omega-3 fatty acids:

- Anchovies
- Bluefish
- Carp
- Catfish
- Halibut
- Herring
- Lake trout
- Mackerel
- Pompano
- Salmon
- Tuna
- Improve fat utilization with 2 to 4 grams a day of L-Carnitine (prescription Carnitor).
- Increase your HDL (the good cholesterol) if it's low with Niacin 5500-1500 per day. Start with lower dose to minimize "flushing" and take an aspirin 20 min before (Niaspan is the prescription grade)
- Maximize soluble fiber (see below).
- If everything else fails to lower your cholesterol and triglycerides, use prescription lipid lowering agents (statins, fibrates, etc).
- If you take lipid lowering drugs, don't forget to take 300 mg a day of Coenzyme Q10 since it has been shown to be low in those taking those medications. This supplement can protect the heart and muscle tissue from damage.
- Take an 81mg baby aspirin a day (with your doctor's approval).

Nutritional Tips:

- Shop mostly in the outer part of the grocery store where the fresh produce, meats, and milk products/eggs are.
- Do not skip breakfast (keep an eye on sugar and refined flour products!)
- Try to eat several smaller meals or snacks instead of two to three large ones.
- Eat more almonds, walnuts, pecans and pistachios (good cholesterol lowering fats).
- Eat fruits and vegetables of all colors.

- Avoid sodas, sweet drinks and fruits juices (fruit sounds healthy but the juice part brings in too many sugars).
- Drink lots of water.
- Eat a high protein, complex carbohydrate- rich meal after work outs.
- Minimize caffeine (it reduces appetite but can increase anxiety).
- Get a slow cooker so that you come back from work to a warm meal.
- Cook for the week and freeze in individual serving sized containers.
- Reduce saturated (animal) fats, fried foods and hydrogenated oils.
- Use good fats: olive oil, nuts, avocados, flaxseed.
- Minimize sugars like fructose (sweets, sodas, and many processed foods are high in fructose corn syrup).
- Eat adequate amounts (0.7-1 gm/lb/day) of protein (fish, eggs, cottage cheese, lean meats, chicken, whey, yogurt, nuts, etc).
- Eat more high-fiber, nutrient and fluid-rich, low calorie, low glycemic carbs like: Oatmeal, multi-grain breads, vegetables, fruits, roots, greens, wild rice and beans.
- Grocery shopping list:
  - Almonds and other nuts
  - Beans and other legumes
  - Spinach and other green leafy vegetables
  - Low fat dairy, yogurt (Greek style)
  - Hummus
  - Whey protein (I like the Isopure brand since it does not give me gut problems and it is very light)
  - Oatmeal (not the little packets; those are loaded with sugars)
  - Eggs (free range or Omega 3 enriched if possible)
  - Lean meats
  - Whole grain breads and pasta
  - Peanut, almond, cashew butters
  - Olive oil and avocados
  - Raspberries and all berries. Whole fruits (remember, not juices)
  - Occasional glass of red wine per day (optional)
  - Flaxseed, pumpkin and sunflower seeds
  - Sweet potatoes and wild rice
  - Green tea

General Exercise Suggestions:

There is controversy in the literature about the effects of exercise on testosterone blood levels. Conflicting results may be explained by differences in the intensity and duration of the activity and the physical characteristics of the individual (e.g. age and fitness level).

Relatively short duration intense activity may lead to transient increases in testosterone concentrations. Athletes who train intensively may experience reductions in testosterone levels but not below normal clinical range. This is not necessarily a consistent phenomenon.

The important thing to remember is that when done correctly, exercise can have the following proven benefits that go beyond just looking good:

- Improved muscle function and strength.
- Reduced trunk (belly) fat
- Increased muscle mass
- Decreased LDL (bad cholesterol).
- Decreased triglycerides. Muscle hypertrophy (enlargement) induced by resistance training, may decrease triglycerides in those with high levels.
- Improved mood and decreased stress.
- Increase bone density in men and women.
- Improved aerobic function and lung capacity.

Getting Started

There are some things to consider before you start an exercise program.. Get your blood pressure, heart rate, weight, body dimensions, fasting cholesterol, triglycerides, and blood sugar measured. Your doctor should be able to advise you if you are capable of exercising without health risks.

If you feel too tired and weak, start by walking every day to your best ability. Walking can increase your energy levels so you can start a more intensive exercise program as you feel better. Use a cheap pedometer to measure your daily steps; try to reach 10,000 steps a day since that amount has been associated with good cardiovascular health and fat loss.

There are two types of exercise: resistance (weight) training and cardiovascular (aerobic) exercise. Resistance training uses weights to induce muscle growth. Cardiovascular exercise improves your body's aerobic capacity (the way it uses oxygen). It also increases your metabolism so that you can burn fat, lower your bad cholesterol and triglycerides, and lower your blood sugar.

Do low-impact aerobic exercise for 20-40 minutes, three to four times a week. Exercises like walking fast, bike riding (stationary or the two-wheeler), stair stepping, and using an elliptical trainer or treadmill are all effective. Switching between different exercises can help keep your interest going. Be careful about aerobic exercise if you are losing weight involuntarily, if you are overly tired or recovering from illness.

Recommendations

Train with weights and machines three times a week for no more than one hour. Starting with machines is the safest way until you get familiar with the exercises. As you feel more confident and strong, bring in free weight exercise (hopefully with the help of a workout buddy). As you get stronger, increase your weights in every exercise. Exercise one body part per week, and do three exercises per body part. One light warm-up set and two heavier sets of eight to ten repetitions to momentary muscle failure (until you cannot do another rep) are enough for each exercise. If you do not have access to a gym, do push-ups on the floor and squats holding books or large bottles full of water at home. As long as you are "resisting" your own body weight, you are doing resistance exercise. You can also get an exercise ball and follow this great home-based workout:
www.myfit.ca/exercisedatabase/search.asp?muscle=Home&
equipment=yes.

For examples of other exercises you can do at home, visit:
weboflife.nasa.gov/exerciseandaging/chapter4_strength.html
For great resistance exercises at the gym,
visit: www.myfit.ca/exercisedatabase/weight_lifting_exercises.asp.

Important Things to Remember

- Learn how to do each exercise correctly. Concentrate on using strict form to get the most out of each exercise and to prevent injuries.
- Make sure your muscles are warm before targeting them with more challenging weights. Warm them up with a light, high-repetition exercise set.

- Don't use your body to add momentum; cheating this way takes work away from the targeted muscles. Use a deliberate speed to increase the effectiveness of the movement.
- Use a full range of motion on all exercises. Feel the muscle stretch at the bottom and go for a momentary peak contraction at the top. Don't go too fast!
- Warm up before you work out and stretch afterwards to prevent injury. Briefly stretch the major muscle groups before your training. This helps flexibility and muscle recovery. For stretching routines,go to: weboflife.nasa.gov/exerciseandaging/chapter4_stretching.html
- Feel the muscles working by keeping your head in what you're doing. Focus on your muscles contracting and relaxing. Concentrate on your body exercising, not on random thoughts or people around you.
- If the weight is too light (more than 12 repetitions), try using a heavier one or do the movement more slowly and really feel the contraction. You should be barely able to finish the tenth rep if your weight is the right one. Of course, as you get stronger with time, increase your weights.
- Keep rest periods to no more than about 20-30 seconds, or shorter, depending on how tired you are from your last set. This will also help to give your heart a mini-workout.

Safety First

Always remember -- safety first! If something you do in an exercise hurts, stop! Ask for help to figure out what you're doing wrong. Maybe it's improper form. If you hurt yourself, you will hinder your progress because you won't want to work out. Learn proper form! Do not exercise if you feel you are coming down with a cold.

Commit Yourself

If you can afford it, join a gym. If you spend the money, you'll be more likely to stay with it, and consistency is the key to success in any exercise program. Also, try to find someone who is enthusiastic to train with, or get a personal trainer (if you can afford one). It's easier to stay motivated when you train with someone else who has a vital interest in your mutual success. It's also safer to have someone to spot you when you lift heavy weight.

Avoid Overtraining

Working out for more than an hour can cause overtraining which can destroy your muscles and decrease your strength. Overtraining is probably the factor most ignored by exercise enthusiasts. Prolonged exercise (overtraining) may lead to suppression of testosterone levels, possibly lasting up to several days.

In order to build muscle the body has to receive a stimulus, a reason, to grow bigger (hypertrophy). It's really very simple: the body only does what it needs to do, what it is required to do. It isn't going to suddenly expand its muscle mass because it anticipates needing more muscles. But if it is challenged to move weights around, it will respond by growing.

Another way to look at it is, if you take any body builder and put him in bed for weeks at a time, he'll begin to rapidly lose muscle mass because the body will sense that it doesn't need the extra muscle any more. By lifting weights one delivers the needed stimulus to begin muscular hypertrophy.

However, overdoing exercise stresses out the body and actually initiates the process of breaking down muscle mass as the body begins to burn its own muscles to use for fuel. This overtraining is why so many people don't grow at a satisfying rate. Even worse, these same people often will think they aren't training hard enough. They *increase* their exercise routines, thinking they just need more stimuli! And this is where the biggest error is made -- more is *not* necessarily better! It seems paradoxical that you could work out *less* and grow *more*, but this is very often the case.

Any exercise beyond that which is the exact amount of stimulus necessary to induce optimal muscle growth is called overtraining. I know this sounds non-specific but the idea is that it will vary from person to person. You need to listen to your body.

A Workout Log Is Recommended

The best reason to keep track of your workouts is so that you can see graphically what you are accomplishing. You will be able to see whether you're gaining strength at a reasonable rate. You can also analyze your pattern to see if you're overtraining. You will find when you log your workouts, that if you are overtraining, you won't be gaining in strength or muscle size. Document your workouts by keeping track of the weight you lift and the amount of reps you lift for each exercise. Then when you go in to train again the next week, you'll know what you are trying to improve upon. If you find out that you're weaker than you were the time before, and everything else like nutrition, etc. is in line, you may be training too often. For downloading workout logs, visit:

www.exrx.net/WeightTraining/WorkoutLogs.html

Food and Hydration

Drink at least eight glasses of water a day to keep hydrated. Dehydration can rob you of energy for your workouts. Drink plenty of water while working out. Avoid sugary drinks, since they will cause fatigue after an initial burst of energy. Some people like to drink green tea or creatine supplements in water before a workout to help increase energy levels through a workout.

A light carbohydrate meal (fruits, carbohydrate drinks, etc.) before a workout and a protein-rich one afterwards is advisable. Keep yourself well hydrated with plenty of water throughout the workout. And get plenty of rest afterwards.

Do not work out right after eating a regular meal; wait at least two hours. If you need a snack, have some fruit and a slice of toast with peanut butter one hour or more before working out. Do not consume protein shakes before working out (leave them for after the workout). Digestion will slow down your workouts and bring your energy down. Within 30-60 minutes after the workout, feed your muscles with a balanced meal containing protein, good fats (olive oil, flaxseed oil), and complex carbohydrates, like fruits and whole grains.

Supplements like glutamine, creatine, and whey protein may be a good thing to consider. A shake containing one heaping tablespoon of glutamine, two tablespoons of Omega 3 oils, one or two scoops of whey protein, some fruit, and milk (if you are lactose intolerant try almond or rice milk, though not soy, since it may increase estrogen in both men and women), provides a good balanced meal after a workout.

Home Based Economical Exercise Helpers

I love the following three cheap devices:

1- An exercise (medicine) ball and elastic bands. You can get one at $14 at Target or any retail store. Make sure it comes with its own pump

You can use these work outs: www.myfit.ca/exercisedatabase/search. asp?muscle=Ball&equipment=yes

2-I love the chin-up (pull-up) bars that you can install on door frames. Here is one that you do not have to install and you can move around: www.amazon.com/Creative-Fitness-DG-Door-Gym/dp/B00029A7C0

3- Get yourself a cheap pedometer in any store to make sure you wear it from the moment you wake up until you go to bed. Ensure that you reach close to 10,000 steps a day for best aerobic capacity. I like the Omron-HJ-150-Hip-pedometer available at amazon.com

Exercise Resources

Two of the best websites for video clips of exercises and an explanation of anatomy are:

www.exrx.net/Lists/Directory.html and www.myfit.ca

Also, several exercise routines are provided on our website, www.medibolics.com/exercise.html

You can also find most exercise routines explained in videos on youtube.com and menshealth.com

-7-

Testosterone Replacement, Side Effects and Management

Interview With
Dr. Michael Scally

Nelson Vergel (NV): Dr. Michael Scally is a well-known expert on men's health in general, and specifically he's an expert on hormone therapy and issues surrounding testosterone replacement. Dr. Scally, can you tell us a little bit about your background?

Michael Scally (MS): My education includes a double degree major in chemistry (1975) and life sciences (1975) from the Massachusetts Institute of Technology (MIT) Cambridge, MA. From 1975 to 1980, in the MIT division of Brain Sciences & Neuroendocrinology, I researched and published investigations on neurotransmitter relationships. During this time, I entered the prestigious Health Sciences & Technology Program, a collaboration of the MIT and Harvard Medical School. In 1980, I was awarded by Harvard Medical School a Doctorate of Medicine, MD. In 1983, I completed a fellowship in anesthesiology at Parkland Southwest Memorial, in Dallas. From 1983 to 1994, I was a private practice anesthesiologist. In 1984, I set up the first ambulatory, outpatient, surgery center at Houston.

In 1994, I became interested in general and preventative medicine with a focus on endocrinology. I have been active in this area since that time.

In 1995, I inquired to Wyeth Pharmaceuticals about the association between primary pulmonary hypertension and pondimin (fenfluramine). I came to learn, this inquiry later was used as evidence in the class-action suit against Wyeth and was instrumental in showing that the known adverse effects were known to Wyeth but not revealed to the public.

During 1994, I competed in the Mr. Texas Bodybuilding Championship, placing second. While exercising, I was approached by a number of weightlifters on the medical treatment to restore the hypothalamic-pituitary axis (HPTA) after stopping anabolic steroids (AAS). Many of these same individuals also used over-the-counter (OTC) supplements.

As you might know, many bodybuilders are trying to decrease their body fat and increase their muscle mass as much as they can. And with these two specific goals in their mind, they were having a hard time because they were taking this over-the-counter supplement. Within a short time later, I discovered an over-the-counter weight loss supplement containing an ingredient, tiratricol, toxic to the thyroid. The reporting of this to the federal agency, MedWatch, was instrumental in the nationwide seizure of the supplement thus avoiding a disaster to the public health and welfare. We published our findings in the peer-reviewed literature, being the first to do so.

This spurred on my interest in the field of men's health, particularly in the field of testosterone and anabolic steroids. I recognized the use of a treatment for stopping anabolic steroids, both prescription and nonprescription, was without any scientific support. The accepted standard of care within the medical community for anabolic steroid-induced hypogonadism is to do nothing with the expectation the individual will return to normal unassisted. This is proving not to be the case and now jeopardizes the health and welfare of countless individuals.

I developed a treatment for anabolic steroid-induced hypogonadism that has been published and presented before the Endocrine Society, the American Association of Clinical Endocrinologists, American College of Sports Medicine, and the International Workshop on Adverse Drug Reactions and Lipodystrophy in HIV. The condition of anabolic steroid-induced hypogonadism is found in nonprescription and prescription AAS alike. The failure of the medical community to recognize the importance of anabolic steroid-induced hypogonadism, particularly in the research setting, is the focus of my recently published book, "Anabolic Steroids—A Question of Muscle: Human Subject Abuses in Anabolic Steroid Research."

NV: There are lots of misconceptions when it comes to testosterone replacement in men. Will you tell us, in your opinion, what are the main misconceptions? For instance, some doctors may think that giving testosterone to somebody with low testosterone may affect the liver, or may cause cancer of the liver or prostate.

MS: There are many misconceptions regarding anabolic steroids, which include testosterone. You mentioned two of the areas: liver and prostate cancer. Other areas are enlargement of the prostate or benign prostate hypertrophy, anabolic steroid dependency, cardiovascular disease, and addiction.

I believe that many of the misconceptions come about by the politicization of anabolic steroids. As far as prescribed medicines are concerned, anabolic steroids are the only group of drugs with a law specifically aimed at their use. This has led to a lack or absence of good research. Instead, what the medical community has relied on are anecdotal and inflammatory reports.

This is probably most evident in the medical community's steadfast refusal to accept that anabolic steroids increase muscle mass and strength. We now know that anabolic steroids conclusively do increase muscle mass and strength and athletic performance.

As far as liver effects, use of the oral anabolic steroids has been reported to cause liver dysfunction and cancer. These reports are primarily in individuals with a preexisting condition treated for extended periods. The intramuscular injections and transdermal preparations do not appear to be associated with liver problems, and routine monitoring is therefore unnecessary. In the thousands of patients I have treated with testosterone, I never even think about liver problems being a contraindication, because they just do not come up.

In non-obstructive benign prostatic hyperplasia (BPH), testosterone replacement therapy is not a concern. The prostate volumes increase in an inconsistent manner. As with any treatment, careful monitoring will alert one to a problem.

As far as prostatic cancer, there is no association. In 2004, a *New England Journal of Medicine* article review of over 60 studies on testosterone replacement therapy concluded that there is no causal or association with prostate cancer.

NV: But testosterone replacement seems to be getting more and more mainstream. Ever since the introduction of gels like Androgel and Testim, more and more doctors feel comfortable prescribing testosterone. But yet, there are still a lot of fears, too. Another fear is changes in lipids and cardiovascular risks associated with testosterone. Can you expand on that a little?

MS: The available data indicate that testosterone replacement therapy within the physiologic range by transdermal or injectable testosterone preparation is not associated with worsening of the lipid profile. Studies using physiologic replacement doses of testosterone show no change, or only a slight decrease, in HDL, often with a reduction in total cholesterol. The oral non-aromatizable anabolic steroids appear to lower high-density lipoprotein (HDL) levels.

The belief that testosterone is a risk factor for cardiac disease is based on the observation that men have both a higher incidence of cardiovascular events and higher testosterone levels than women do. There is little data for this idea. Many studies suggest the opposite. There are multiple studies showing a relation between hypogonadism and an increased cardiovascular risk.

There is evidence that testosterone replacement therapy may be beneficial for men with cardiac disease. In a small study, men with chronic stable angina who were treated with transdermal testosterone replacement therapy had greater angina free exercise tolerance. Importantly, testosterone replacement therapy has not shown an increased incidence of cardiovascular disease or stroke.

NV: There are some data on hypogonadism and increased risks of cardiovascular events. Is that what you mean? Some people actually become so severely hypogonadal, they actually may be risking higher incidence of heart attacks and strokes?

MS: That is correct. There are numerous studies demonstrating the relationship between low testosterone levels and adverse cardiovascular events, as well as stroke. Also, there are case study reports of people who stop anabolic steroids, and then suffer a heart attack.

In the book that I wrote, one of the studies in the published literature, looking at the effects of anabolic steroids in certain populations, for 12 weeks, did not look at the patients after they stopped the drug. If you want to look at the effects of these drugs, you need to see what happens when you stop them. I filed a Freedom of Information Act to obtain the patient records. One of the patients actually suffered a heart attack within four weeks of stopping the anabolic steroid. The details, including the original patient records, of this case are reported in my book.

NV: Should patients with an increased or elevated prostatic specific antigen (PSA) avoid testosterone? What role does testosterone

replacement therapy (TRT) have on prostate cancer, if any? Is there a risk of worsening prostate cancer with TRT?

MS: You brought up a number of important and controversial issues. It is generally agreed that TRT with established prostate cancer is contra-indicated.

It is known that suppression of testosterone levels causes regression of prostate cancer, and it is now commonplace for men with metastatic prostate cancer to undergo treatment designed to lower testosterone levels. The question becomes if lowering testosterone causes prostate cancer to regress, does elevating testosterone cause prostate cancer to appear?

There are case reports suggesting that TRT may convert an occult cancer into a clinically apparent lesion. These studies are wrong. One must be very careful in attributing causality to testosterone, since over 200,000 men are given a diagnosis of prostate cancer each year, and most of these cases are first detected by a rise in the PSA level unrelated to testosterone therapy. Studies have demonstrated a low frequency of prostate cancer in association with TRT. Despite extensive research, there is no compelling evidence that testosterone has a causative role in prostate cancer.

There appears to be no compelling evidence at present to suggest that men with higher testosterone levels are at greater risk of prostate cancer or treating men who have hypogonadism with exogenous androgens increases this risk. In fact, prostate cancer becomes more prevalent exactly at the time of a man's life when testosterone levels decline.

Little evidence exists on the safety of TRT initiation after treatment for primary prostate cancer. In one very small case series, TRT after treatment of organ confined prostate cancer produced no adverse effects. There are no large, long-term studies proving that the risk of recurrence is not affected by TRT. Personally, I would be reluctant to provide TRT in prostate cancer; treatment should be left to strict research protocols.

PSA is a serum glycoprotein made by the normal prostate that is widely used as a tumor marker, because elevated PSA levels correlate with the risk of prostate cancer. A PSA value greater than 4.0 ng/mL has been the standard indication for prostate biopsy since the introduction of this test in the 1980s.

Testosterone trials have inconsistently shown a rise in PSA, typically between 0.2 and 0.5 ng/mL. A greater increase in PSA arouses concern that prostate cancer has developed. It is my practice to recommend a prostate biopsy in any patient with a yearly PSA increase of 1.0 ng/mL or more. If the PSA level increases by 0.75 ng/mL in one year, I repeat the PSA measurement in three to six months and recommend a biopsy if there is any further increase.

NV: Can you explain what polycythemia is and what it means when it comes to cardiovascular risk and other issues?

MS: In respect to anabolic steroid-induced polycythemia, polycythemia is a condition that results in an increased level of circulating red blood cells in the blood stream. Erythrocytosis is a more specific term that is used to denote increased red blood cells. People with polycythemia have an increase in hematocrit, hemoglobin, or red blood cell count above the normal limits. The reporting of polycythemia is typically in terms of increased hematocrit or hemoglobin.

Hematocrit is a blood test that measures the percentage of red blood cells found in the whole blood. This measurement depends on the number and size of red blood cells. Normally, for a male, the hematocrit raises up to a level of 52–54 depending on the reporting laboratory reference range. Polycythemia is considered when the hematocrit is greater than the upper limit of normal.

Hemoglobin is the protein molecule in red blood cells that carries oxygen from the lungs to the body's tissues and returns carbon dioxide from the tissues to the lungs. The hemoglobin level is expressed as the amount of hemoglobin in grams (g) per deciliter (dl) of the whole blood, a deciliter being 100 mL, for adult males: 14–18 gm/dL. Polycythemia is considered when a hemoglobin level is greater than 18 g/dL in men.

It is a thickening of the blood. The blood becomes almost like sludge. You would think that with the increased number of red blood cells, it would carry more oxygen; but its oxygen-carrying capacity decreases markedly. Without treatment, polycythemia can be life threatening. Elevation above the normal range may have grave consequences, particularly in the elderly, since an attendant increase in blood viscosity could aggravate vascular disease in the coronary, cerebrovascular, or peripheral vascular circulation. However, with proper medical care, many people experience few problems related to this disease.

Symptoms of polycythemia can be none to minimal in many people. Some general and nonspecific symptoms include weakness, fatigue, headache, itching, redness of your skin, bruising, joint pain, dizziness, abdominal pain, shortness of breath, breathing difficulty when you lie down; and numbness, tingling, or burning in the hands, feet, arms, or legs.

NV: Or when they work out, they turn purple.

MS: That can certainly be a symptom of polycythemia.

NV: Is the incidence of polycythemia related to the route of administration, dose, duration, and age? Is polycythemia common in replacement doses?

MS: Yes. It occurs quite frequently in people who are just on replacement testosterone. Older men appear more sensitive to the erythropoietic effects of testosterone than young men do. Both testosterone dose and mode of delivery affect the magnitude of hematocrit elevation.

The incidence of testosterone-associated polycythemia may be lower in males receiving pharmacokinetically steady-state delivery of testosterone formulations, than it is in receiving intramuscular injections.

In patients using topical preparations, there is a 5–20 percent incidence of erythrocytosis. There is an apparent direct relation between testosterone dosage and the incidence of erythrocytosis. Erythrocytosis occurs in about 5–15 percent by patches and in 10–20 percent with gel preparations depending on the use of 50 mg/day (delivering 5 mg /day) and 100 mg/day (delivering 10 mg/day) during the course of approximately 14 year.

The most commonly used forms of intramuscular-injectable testosterone esters are testosterone enanthate and cypionate. Injectable testosterone esters generate supranormal testosterone levels shortly after injection and then testosterone levels decline very rapidly, becoming subnormal in the days before the next injection.

Testosterone ester injections have been reported to be associated with a higher risk of erythrocytosis than transdermal testosterone. It is unclear whether the higher frequency of erythrocytosis observed with injectable testosterone esters is due to the higher dose of testosterone delivered by the injections or the higher peaks of testosterone levels. In one study, intramuscular injections of testosterone enanthate produced an elevated hematocrit over 40 percent.

NV: Is therapeutic phlebotomy a good way to manage polycythemia?

MS: Untoward events are unlikely with mild erythrocytosis of relatively short duration. Therapeutic phlebotomy and blood donation are overall a safe procedure, the frequency of side effects being low and their severity weak. Other options include dosage reduction or the withholding of testosterone. However, these latter options can be problematic since the patient will experience symptoms of anabolic steroid-induced hypogonadism.

This does present a catch-22 for many physicians. Because the half-life of the red blood cell is approximately 120 days, it might be a considerable length of time, more than three months or longer, to normalize the hemoglobin or hematocrit upon TRT cessation. But, the problem of anabolic steroid-induced hypogonadism symptoms complicated matters.

Many a times, an attempt will be to maintain TRT while simultaneously performing a therapeutic phlebotomy. Because of the increased erythropoiesis, production of red blood cells, it feels like the proverbial chasing one's tail. In a number of therapeutic phlebotomies, the units of the blood that have to be taken off are clearly quite excessive; and we do not want to do that too quickly. It may come to be three, four, or even five pints of blood that have to be taken off.

In order to get a good hold on the problem of polycythemia, it will be necessary to discontinue TRT. What we have done again, in our protocol, is that we have stopped the testosterone, thereby removing the cause of the increased red blood cell production, treat them with the HPTA protocol that prevents the hypogonadism, and have the therapeutic phlebotomy done. They are able to get the hemoglobin or hematocrit down to the normal level, do not go through the adverse effects of the hypogonadism; and then, at the other end, be able to start the testosterone therapy again. As far as we can determine, no testosterone associated thromboembolic events have been reported to date.

NV: I am actually surprised how many patients are out there that do not have their physician following up their hematocrit when they are put on testosterone or anabolics for wasting syndrome. It is something that the physician should be looking out for and measuring.

MS: The hemoglobin and hematocrit is part of the routine laboratory follow-up for anyone on TRT. If a patient complains of any of the symptoms we describe for polycythemia, a hemoglobin and hematocrit should be checked. One of the confounding problems is the symptoms tend to be nonspecific.

NV: Can you say something about the prophylactic use of finasteride or dutasteride to avoid DHT-related problems like prostate enlargement

or hair loss? Is there a role for the use of finasteride or dutasteride to prevent the possible increase of hair loss with TRT?

MS: Finasteride and dutasteride are 5-alpha reductase inhibitors. 5-alpha reductase comes in two forms, type 1 and type 2, and is responsible for the conversion of testosterone into DHT. Finasteride inhibits type 2 only while dutasteride inhibits both forms.

Finasteride comes in two doses depending on whether the indication is for hair loss or benign prostate hypertrophy. Propecia, 1 mg, is for hair loss. Proscar, 5 mg, is for prostatic hypertrophy.

DHT has been shown to be important in the development of hair loss or male pattern baldness. I am unaware any studies indicating a worsening of hair loss or male pattern baldness, though this possibility has not been carefully studied. There are anecdotal reports. The prophylactic use of these drugs is an individual decision after weighing the risks and benefits.

DHT is also important in prostate health. It is thought an overabundance of DHT may be important in benign prostatic hyperplasia (BPH) and prostate cancer. Dutasteride provides greater suppression of DHT than finasteride does, thereby underlying the hypothesis that inhibition of both type 1 and type 2 would provide correspondingly greater protection than inhibition of type 2 alone.

However, significant side effects of finasteride use include reduced volume of ejaculate, erectile dysfunction, loss of libido, and gynecomastia. This will prevent many from their use.

Some people think that DHT will affect lean body composition. DHT does have a higher affinity for the androgen receptor. But the enzyme that converts testosterone into DHT is not located in the muscle. There is no evidence for these drugs to effect muscle mass.

NV: What about other issues related TRT, such as to increased estrogen levels and gynecomastia?

MS: A small number report breast tenderness and swelling. Fluid retention is uncommon and generally mild, but TRT should be used cautiously in men with congestive heart failure or renal insufficiency. After confirmation of elevated estrogen, estradiol, levels, this can be treated with either an aromatization inhibitor or estradiol receptor blocker. This must be done very carefully as any prolonged reduction in estradiol levels runs the risk of causing osteoporosis.

Exacerbation of sleep apnea or the development of sleep apnea has been associated with TRT who have other identifiable risk factors for sleep apnea. The mechanism appears to be central mediated rather than by means of changes in the airway. Other side effects include acne, oily skin, increased body hair, and flushing. Hypertension has rarely been reported.

Of course, the adverse effect I am most concerned with is androgen-induced hypogonadism, which occurs in one hundred percent of individuals stopping TRT, the variables being the duration and severity.

On testosterone replacement therapy, for those without organic hypogonadism, those with late onset of hypogonadism, the only thing that I always caution about is that people should not be on testosterone replacement therapy, year after year after year, without stopping every 12–18 months to restore the axis, to make sure the function is still there. The longer you are on testosterone, the harder it is going to be to come off testosterone.

NV: In your opinion, can you tell us a little bit about the different options for TRT? Have you seen any difference in using gels versus injections? Is there any advantage or disadvantage to using either one?

MS: Injectable, transdermal, buccal, and oral testosterone formulations are available for clinical use. These forms of treatment differ in several key areas.

Oral preparations include methyltestosterone and fluoxymesterone, which are rarely prescribed because of their association with substantial liver toxicity. In Europe, there is an oral preparation of testosterone undecenoate, Andriol. It has a poor history of bioavailability.

Recently, the FDA approved a buccal preparation of testosterone, Striant. Striant requires administration twice a day. It is used little at this time.

Transdermal testosterone is available as a patch, Testim, and gel, Androgel. Daily application is required for each of these. They are designed to deliver 5–10 mg of testosterone a day. The advantages include ease of use and maintenance of relatively uniform serum testosterone levels over time. Skin irritation in the form of itching and redness is a frequent adverse effect of Testim with reports as high as 60–70 percent. This is uncommon with Androgel. Inadequate absorption through the skin may limit the value of transdermal preparations in some persons. A common problem is the low dose preparations provide inadequate serum testosterone levels. This is also seen with the high dose.

The topicals have become, by far, the most-used products in the last decade or so, approaching a billion dollars in sales. Androgel is the biggest product of the topicals.

If the patient is not too scared of doing injectables, oil-based testosterone ester preparations are available. The most commonly used injectables are Delatestryl or testosterone enanthate and depo testosterone or testosterone cypionate. In my practice, the typical dose is between 100 and 150 mg/week. The peak serum levels occur in 2–5 days after injection, and a return to baseline is usually observed 10 days after injection. In this manner, adequate serum levels are maintained. Intramuscular injections of testosterone can cause local pain, soreness, bruising, redness, swelling, and possible infection.

NV: Most doctors prescribe 1-cc of 200 mL of testosterone every two weeks. Can you describe the problems with this schedule, if any?

MS: This is a problem that is seen much more often than necessary. Many doctors use a typical dose is 100 mg/week, or 200–300 mg every two to three weeks.

Within 7–10 days after injection, the serum testosterone levels are low to abnormally low. This is described as a "roller coaster" effect, characterized by alternating periods of symptomatic benefit and a return to baseline symptoms, corresponding to the fluctuations in serum testosterone levels. This can be discovered by having the testosterone level checked within 24 hours prior to injection.

NV: Can you talk to us a little bit about compounding pharmacy products? In particular, when using testosterone gels with concentrations higher than 1 percent for reaching total testosterone blood levels above 500 ng/L. Have you had any experience with the compounding industry?

MS: I have had some experience with the compounding industry. Compounding pharmacies are very capable at providing higher concentrations of transdermal testosterone preparations. Because of this, they are able to supply a transdermal product in small volumes. They also tend to be less expensive than commercially available pharmaceutical testosterone replacement options.

NV: Do you think it is advisable to get your testosterone levels re-checked after a few weeks of starting any of the therapies?

MS: My protocol is that once I start a patient on testosterone, I check the testosterone level 4–6 weeks after initiating TRT. In patients using topical preparations, I recommend testing within 4–6 hours after application. Those using injectables of testosterone esters, I recommend testing within 24 hours before their next scheduled injection.

NV: Do you have any preference between the free testosterone and total testosterone test?MS: In the monitoring of the patient on TRT, I utilize the total testosterone. The initial evaluation of a patient might include the use of free testosterone or bioavailable testosterone. In a symptomatic individual, the total testosterone can be normal but the free or bioavailable testosterone abnormal.

Testosterone circulates in three forms. Testosterone circulates in a free or unbound state, tightly bound to SHBG, or weakly bound to the blood protein albumin. Bioavailable, non-SHBG, testosterone includes free testosterone and testosterone that is bound to albumin but does not include SHBG -bound testosterone.

Examined changes over time have demonstrated a decrease in the total testosterone and an increase in SHBG levels. Because of this, the total testosterone might be normal, whereas the free or bioavailable testosterone is abnormal. If these alternative methods are used to diagnose hypogonadism, their utility during TRT is limited.

I would caution about the assay methodology used to calculate the free or bioavailable testosterone. The methods used to conduct the measurements vary in their accuracy, standardization, the extent of validation, and the reproducibility of results.

Bioavailable testosterone is measured or calculated in several ways. SHBG bound testosterone can be precipitated with ammonium sulfate and the remaining testosterone is then taken as the bioavailable.

Measures of free testosterone (FT) are controversial. The only standardized and validated method is equilibrium dialysis or by calculating free testosterone levels based on separate measurements of testosterone and SHBG. Other measures of free testosterone are less accurate.

NV: And your goal is usually to have patients above what level?

MS: I like their total testosterone trough or lower level to be in the 500–700 range, normal being 300–1,000 ng/dL.

NV: Besides checking of the initial T level, can you elaborate on the monitoring during TRT?

I recommend a periodic follow-up of patients receiving replacement testosterone therapy at the interval of three months during the first year of treatment.

Afterward, patients are followed up every six months. It is important to do a review of systems to ensure the relief of the complaining symptoms as well as no worsening or new symptoms.

In addition to the serum total testosterone, I routinely monitor the basic chemistry profile, which includes liver function, kidney function, electrolytes, glucose, lipid panel, and hemoglobin or hematocrit. At three months, I will often include estradiol and DHT levels.

If the patient is older than 50 years, I include the PSA. The role of digital rectal examination (DRE) and PSA in detecting early, clinically significant, prostate cancer is controversial. I discuss this with each patient and allow them to decide on their use.

NV: How about the new non-steroidal androgens that are in the pipeline? Can you tell us what you have read about them?

MS: They are called SARM: selective androgen receptor modulators. They are going to become more and more popular. The closest SARM that is coming to the market, and it is years away, is called ostarine. It is being developed by GTx, Inc. Ligand Pharmaceuticals has a SARM in early phase of development. They are both traded on the NASDAQ Exchange.

The initial studies are being done in cancer patients. The data collected is change in muscle mass and strength. The clinical outcome being measured is the six-minute walk test.

My feeling on this is that we have a long way to go before these things come to market. If they come to market within the next 5–10 years, we will be lucky. As far as I know, these are the only SARMs in human clinical trials.

NV: I have also heard that SARMs may not have any influence on sexual function, only on lean body mass and maybe some functional capacity. They are really not replacement of testosterone. Are they?

MS: From the initial studies, these are meant to take the place of anabolic steroids, not testosterone. There are no indications SARMs are being developed as TRT. The data from both animal and human studies is that they act similarly, if not identically, to anabolic steroids. They act through the androgen receptor. They do cause HPTA suppression.

Even though they have the same effect, they will be able to be marketed without that name "anabolic steroids." This would be an obvious advantage in their marketing. It should be noted that these drugs, SARMs, have already found their way into the nonprescription or illicit market.

NV: Can somebody on testosterone replacement become less fertile? If a man wants to impregnate his wife after, let us say, a year of testosterone replacement, is there any risk for that man to become less fertile to his wife?

MS: Testicular size and consistency often diminish, and men should be advised that fertility would be greatly compromised during testosterone replacement therapy because of downregulation of LH and FSH.

The general rule is they will become less fertile. But you cannot depend on its use as a fertility drug. And that is where we come in with contraceptive studies. We have many, many contraceptive studies that use testosterone cypionate at 200 mg a week and find that, yes, it decreases fertility. But there is still a subset of men that still produce sperm that are fertile.

NV: Are these men good candidates for a protocol to reset their HPGA?

MS: We have had many men who come to the clinic with the actual complaint that they were using anabolic steroids, or they were using testosterone, and they now want to get their wife pregnant. Although many will return to normal after stopping TRT, this period can be lengthy.

The amazing thing to me is that the number of people that come to me, who have seen the doctor, who are either non-prescription or prescription anabolic steroid users, testosterone with or without combination of anabolic steroids, who have the problem of infertility; and their doctors have no idea what to do, except to do nothing. But on top of this are all the psychological problems and effects that come along with doing nothing as a consequence of anabolic steroid-induced hypogonadism. The HPTA protocol has restored fertility as well as decreased the time substantially.

NV: Can you expand about resetting the HPGA?

The word resetting is a misnomer, though recent studies published in the *New England Journal of Medicine* (NEJM) do indicate this possible. In 2007, the *NEJM* reports on the resetting of the HPTA after TRT for adult onset idio-pathic hypogonadism. This is the first report demonstrating HPTA plasticity in adulthood. The term I prefer is HPTA functionality and restoration.

There are clear conditions under which testosterone requires administration for life-long treatment. However, there are increasing numbers of individuals being treated with TRT who do not fall under these disorders. TRT is being prescribed more and more for late onset hypogonadism. This is called by many other names, including andropause, androgen deficiency of the aging male, and others.

There are no consequences of the decline in serum testosterone with age that are known with certainty. Several parallels exist between the effects of aging and those of hypogonadism, which suggest that the decline in serum testosterone might be a cause of several effects of aging. Since the long-term effects of androgen treatment for late onset hypogonadism or andropause are not well-known, I discontinue therapy on an approximate annual basis to ensure HPTA normalization—functionality. This allows the patient the autonomy to stop therapy should the need arise.

What is clear is that upon stopping testosterone or anabolic steroids, a period of anabolic steroid-induced hypogonadism ensues. This occurs in one hundred percent of individuals stopping testosterone. The only variables are the duration and severity. The duration of hypogonadism, or the severity of hypogonadism, is typically related to the anabolic steroid drug, dose, and duration.

In other words, one person that is on testosterone for an entire year; they may come back to normal within 1 or 2 months. Another person may take 12, 18 months, or even 3 years to come back to normal. The best studies we have on this are contraceptive studies with testosterone for over a year. And what we find in those studies is that it may take up to three years for a person to return to normal.

If they have been taking those anabolic steroids to improve their body composition, increase the lean body mass, and decrease the body fat, that all goes back to normal after stopping anabolic steroids. But you are also going to be exposed to the other adverse effects of hypogonadism, which include adverse psychological and cardiovascular effects. Some of the adverse psychological effects are depression, decreased cognitive abilities, insomnia, decreased libido, and erection dysfunction. More significantly, after cessation adds the comorbid condition of hypogonadism to their already existing chronic illness.

AAS, including testosterone, licit and illicit, administration induces a state of hypogonadism that continues after their cessation. All compounds classified as androgens or anabolic steroids cause a negative feedback inhibition of the hypothalamic-pituitary testicular axis, suppress endogenous gonadotropin secretion, and as a consequence serum testosterone.

The symptoms of AIH are identical to classical hypogonadism. This problem prevents many of discontinuing testosterone or anabolic steroids. As we have said, there are many reasons for stopping testosterone, including polycythemia, gynecomastia, and other issue as compliance, affordability, and changing life style.

The accepted standard of care within the medical community for anabolic steroid induced hypogonadism is to do nothing with the expectation the individual will return to normal unassisted. But the literature shows this not to be the case.

AIH is critical toward any planned use of AAS or similar compound to effect positive changes in muscle mass and muscle strength as well as an understanding for what has been termed anabolic steroid dependency. The further understanding and treatments that mitigate or prevent AIH could contribute to androgen therapies for wasting associated diseases and stopping nonprescription AAS use.

NV: What is used for restoring the hormonal axis?

MS: A combination of three drugs. The individual use of HCG, clomiphene citrate, and tamoxifen is well-known, well-accepted, and well-tested standards of care treatments in peer-reviewed medical literature for diagnostic testing for underlying pathology of hypogonadism. The HPTA protocol uses the medications human chorionic gonadotropin, clomiphene citrate, and tamoxifen.

The first phase of the HPTA protocol examines the functionality of the testicles by the direct action of HCG. HCG raises sex hormone levels directly through the stimulation of the testes and secondly decreases the production and level of gonadotropin LH. The increase in serum testosterone with the HCG stimulation is useful in determining whether any primary testicular dysfunction is present.

This initial value is a measure of the ability of the testicles to respond to stimulation from HCG. Demonstration of the HPTA functionality is an adequate response of the testicles to raise the serum level of T well into the normal range. If this is observed, HCG is discontinued. The failure of the testes to respond to an HCG challenge is indicative of primary testicular failure. In the simplest terms, the first half of the protocol is to determine testicular production and reserve by direct stimulation with HCG. If one is unable to obtain adequate (normal) levels successfully in the first half, there is little cause or reason to proceed to the second half.

The second phase of the HPTA protocol, clomiphene and tamoxifen, examines the ability of the hypothalamic-pituitary axis to respond to stimulation by producing LH levels within the normal reference range. The clomiphene citrate challenge differentiates secondary hypogonadism. Clomiphene is an antiestrogen, which decreases the estrogen effect in the body. It has a dual effect by stimulating the hypothalamic pituitary area and it has an antiestrogenic effect, so that it decreases the effect of estrogen in the body. Tamoxifen is more of a strict antiestrogen, it decreases the effect of estrogen in the body, and potentiates the action of clomiphene. Tamoxifen and clomiphene citrate compete with estrogen for estrogen receptor binding sites, thus eliminating excess estrogen circulation at the level of the hypothalamus and pituitary, allowing gonadotropin production to resume. Administering them together produces an elevation of LH and secondarily gonadal sex hormones. The administration of clomiphene leads to an appropriate rise in the levels of LH, suggesting that the negative feedback control on the hypothalamus is intact and that the storage and release of gonadotropins by the pituitary is normal. If there was a successful stimulation of testicular T levels by HCG, but an inadequate or no response in LH production, then the patient has hypogonadotropic, secondary, hypogonadism.

In the simplest terms, the second half of the protocol is to determine hypothalamo-pituitary production and reserve with clomiphene and tamoxifen. The physiological type of hypogonadism—hypogonadotropic or secondary—is characterized by abnormal low or low normal gonadotropin (LH) production in response to clomiphene citrate and tamoxifen. In the functional type of hypogonadism, the ability to stimulate the HPTA to produce LH and T levels within the normal reference range occurs.

There is a dearth of good studies in anabolic steroids, both while you are taking them and after you stop them, I think this is going to be something that we are going to need to look at in the future. In fact, we are going to plan on looking at it in our proposed clinical studies that we have with our company for the prevention of anabolic steroid-induced hypogonadism.

Dr Michael Scally can be contacted at mscally@alum.mit.edu. His book "Anabolic Steroids - A Question of Muscle: Human Subject Abuses in Anabolic Steroid Research" is available on Amazon.com

-APPENDIX A-

CONFIDENTIAL MEDICAL HISTORY FORM
(Courtesy of Dr John Crisler allthingsmale.com)

WE REALIZE THIS MEDICAL HISTORY FORM IS SOMEWHAT LONG. HOWEVER, IT IS ABSOLUTELY NECESSARY FOR US TO EVALUATE YOUR GENERAL HEALTH AND SAFELY AND LEGITIMATELY PRESCRIBE THE MEDICATIONS YOU WANT AND NEED. MAKE SURE TO TAKE A FEW MINUTES TO CAREFULLY AND COMPLETELY ANSWER EVERY QUESTION. FAILING TO DO SO WILL PREVENT US FROM HELPING YOU, AS DOING SO COULD POSSIBLY JEOPARDIZE YOUR HEALTH. DO THE BEST YOU CAN-WE WILL FOLLOW-UP WITH ANY QUESTIONS WE MAY HAVE. REMEMBER, THIS INFORMATION IS COMPLETELY CONFIDENTIAL.

Please initial here that you have read the above statement: _____

I am a NEW /ESTABLISHED patient (circle one).
Password (established patients only):

1. First name:
2. Middle name:
3. Last name:
4. Address:
5. City:
6. State:
7. Zip code:
8. Shipping address (if different than address above):
9. City:
10. State:
11. Zip code:

CONTACT INFORMATION

12. Email:
13. Repeat Email Address [to confirm]:
14. Daytime phone:
15. Night time phone:

PERSONAL INFORMATION

16. Birth date:
17. Driver's License Number:
18. Social Security Number:
19. Marital Status (Married, Divorced, Never Married, Gay)
20. Sex:
21. Height:
22. Weight:
23. Occupation:
24. Medical Insurance Provider and member ID:
25. Prescription Insurance Provider and member ID:
26. Do you have a primary care physician?
27. When was your last complete physical examination?
28. What were the results of that exam?
29. Will you have a copy of that report and any labs sent to us (mail or FAX)?
30. (FOR OVER 40) Did you have your prostate examined?
31. (FOR OVER 40) Did you have your PSA checked?
If so, what was it?

PAST MEDICAL HISTORY

Please indicate if you now have, or have EVER had:
32. Anemia
33. Arthritis
34. Asthma
35. Blood disease
36. Bronchitis
37. Diabetes
38. Emphysema

39. Epilepsy
40. Gout
41. Hepatitis
42. Heart disease
43. High blood pressure
44. High cholesterol
45. Kidney disease
46. Migraines
47. Mononucleosis
48. Pneumonia
49. Psychological problems
50. Rheumatic fever
51. Seizures
52. Stroke
53. Thyroid disease
54. TB
55. Ulcers
56. Urinary tract infections
57. Have you ever had any form of cancer?
If so, please detail:

PAST SURGICAL HISTORY

What surgeries have you had?

58. Appendectomy
59. Cholecystectomy (gall bladder removal)
60. Mastectomy (removal of breast material-usually for gynocomastia)
61. Tonsillectomy
62. Prostatectomy
63. Hernia repair
64. Other surgeries (please explain):

65. Have you ever been hospitalized (other than for the above mentioned surgeries)?

If so, please list the reason and give approximate date(s):

FAMILY MEDICAL HISTORY

Have your brothers and/or sisters, parents or grandparents, ever had (Please tell which family member(s)?
66. Heart attack
67. Diabetes
68. Kidney disease
69. Leukemia
70. Mental disorders
71. Stroke
72. Prostate cancer
73. Other cancer
Please detail ANY of the above:

74. Are you allergic to anything?
75. If yes, what?

76. Do you smoke?
77. If so, how much each day?
78. How long have you smoked?
79. Do you drink alcohol?
How many drinks do you typically have in a week?

80. Do you use any illicit substances (get high)?
If so, which ones?

REVIEW OF SYSTEMS

Do you CURRENTLY have (please circle)?:
81.   Head aches

82. Vision changes
83. Hearing changes
84. Chronic sinusitis
85. Allergic sinus problems
86. Any tenderness or sores in your mouth or throat
87. Bloody noses
88. Chronic cough
89. Do you spit up blood?
90. Shortness of breath
91. Chest pain
92. Dizziness
93. Congestive heart failure
94. Palpitations
95. Any form of arrythmia
96. Heart murmur
97. Recurring constipation
98. Recurring diarrhea
99. Gallbladder disease
100. Throw up blood
101. Blood in your stool or black tarry stool
102. Hernia
103. Loss of appetite
104. Indigestion
105. Nausea
106. Vomiting
107. Jaundice (yellow skin)
108. Do your eyes look yellow?
109. Do you have abdominal pain?
If so, please describe and tell where:

110. Pancreatitis
111. Do you urinate alright?
112. Does it hurt when you urinate?
113. Is there any blood in your urine?
114. Have you ever had a STD (Sexually Transmitted Disease)?
115. Tingling in your fingers or toes
116. Acne

Describe any acne history:

117. Do you ever pass out?
118. Do you have cold intolerance?
119. Do you bruise easily?
120. Depression
121. Anxiety
122. Decreased sexual potency
If so, is this causing stress in your relationship?

123. Sleep disturbances
124. Generalized muscle aches and pains
125. Joint pain
126. Back pain
127. Fatigue
128. Lethargy
129. Nocturnal emissions
130. Sensitive or swollen nipples?
131. Did you have swollen or painful nipples BEFORE you ever used steroids (for Steroid Consult only)?
132. Can you feel any lumps around your nipples
133. Are you losing your hair?
Were you losing it before you started using steroids (AAS Consult only)?
If so, is it falling out more quickly now?

GENERAL

134. Loss of appetite
135. Unexplained weight loss
136. Do you consider yourself to be in good health?
137. Do you sleep well?
Average hours of sleep per night:

138. Do you regularly self examine your testicles?
139. Tell me about your diet (Details please)

MEDICATIONS

140. Do you take any prescription medications (other than steroids)? If so, please list, and give dosages:

141. What supplements do you take (vitamins, minerals, neutraceuticals, etc.)? List all(with amounts or dosages) each day.

142. How much water do you usually drink each day?

QUESTIONS FOR STEROID CONSULT ONLY (for confidential information only- We do not prescribe these agents for non medical uses)

143. Tell us, as accurately as you can which steroids you are going to take, or have taken, for THIS cycle (AAS Consult only):
144. How many times have you been on a steroid cycle (if any)?
145. How long ago was your first steroid cycle (if any)?
146. How long was your break before starting this cycle?

147. Describe your past usage, if any, of hCG, Nolvadex, Clomid, Arimidex or finasteride:
148. Have you ever had any problems (side effects) with any of the medications mentioned in question #147 If so, please describe:
149. Which of the ancillaries are you looking for, and how much of each do you want (AAS Consult only)? This question is for experienced AAS users only.

HRT patients only (questions 150-159):

150. Do you plan on having more children?
151. Do you have a decrease **in** sex drive?
152. If the answer to #151 is "YES", is this affecting your relationship?
153. Has your strength or endurance decreased?
154. Are you enjoying life less?
155. Are you sad or grumpy?
156. Are your erections less strong?
157. Has your work performance decreased?
158. Do you have a hard time recovering from physical activity?
159. Have you ever been on HRT before?

CONGRATULATIONS! YOU ARE (FINALLY!) DONE WITH THIS FORM.

I HAVE COMPLETED THE MEDICAL HISTORY FORM TO THE BEST OF MY KNOWLEDGE. I CERTIFY THAT MY ANSWERS ARE COMPLETE, HONEST AND TRUE.

Signed: Date: _____

-APPENDIX B-

Resources

Internet Discussion Groups

Subscribe to a yahoo group that discusses testosterone replacement by sending an email to

Hypogonadism2-subscribe@yahoogroups.com

This group exchanges several emails a day about testosterone replacement and erectile dysfunction.

Another good web site to join is: www.mesomorphosis.com. There you can join forums on testosterone, exercise, nutrition, supplements, and other topics related to fitness.

On Facebook, I have created a page called "Testosterone Wisdom". Please search those key words and join us!

I will be posting updates on **TestosteroneWisdom.com** frequently on latest developments in the field and also my own experiences.

Patient Assistance Programs

Testim

If you have insurance but it charges you a high copayment for the drug, you can apply for co-pay assistance. If you have questions about this program please contact the Testim Voucher Hotline at 1-877-217-5737

Testim's copy program is not valid for claims submitted by or on behalf of a patient for reimbursement or coverage for Testim under Medicaid, Medicare, or other federal or state government health care programs. Not valid in conjunction with any 3rd party payor program in Massachusetts.

https://www.trialcard.com/WebRebate/Testim2008/

For men who do not have insurance and meet the financial criteria, the following information can guide them on how to apply for free product.

Program Name	Auxilium Patient Assistance Program
Program Address	40 Valley Stream Parkway Malvem, PA 19355
Phone Number	877-663-0412
Fax Number	866-837-7293
Medications on Program	Testim 1% Gel 1% gel 50 mg (testosterone topical)
Application Forms	Auxilium Patient Assistance Program: www.needymeds.org/papforms/auxili0462.pdf
Online Application	No on-line application available at this time
Eligibility Guidelines and Notes	The patient must have no prescription coverage for the requested medication and have an income at or below $23,660 per individual, $29,140 for 2 people, $36,620 for 3 people, $44,100 for 4 people, etc. The patient must have a diagnosis of hypogonadism. The patient must also reside in the US. Patients must be male. Patients who were eligible for Medicare Part D, but did not enroll may still be eligible for this program. Patients who enrolled in Medicare Part D, but are in the Donut Hole are not eligible. Applicants that do not qualify under the program's set criteria may still apply by completing the "Hardship Exception Request" section of the application form.
Application Process	Anyone requesting assistance can call to request a faxed application or download it from the website. The application will be faxed out. The completed application must be mailed back. The patient is notified of eligibility for the program. The decision is made at meetings that occur approximately every month. (Speak to the company for specifics.) The medication is shipped within 4-6 weeks of receiving the application.
Application Requirements	The doctor must fill out a section, sign the application and attach a prescription for 6 months. The patient must fill out a section, sign the application and attach a denial letter from Medicaid.
Program Details	A six-month supply is sent to the doctor's office. The company automatically sends out refills. Every six months a new application is needed with a new prescription, once a year an application with documentation is needed.

Androgel

If you have insurance but your co-pay is too high, you can apply for a co-pay assistance by visiting: https://webrebate.trialcard.com/coupon/androgelportal/QuizPrescribe.aspx

If you do not have insurance and meet the financial criteria, you can get the product for free. Here is the information to apply:

Program Name	Solvay Pharmaceuticals Patient Assistance Program
Program Address	C/O Express Scripts Speciality Distribution Svc. PO Box 66550 St. Louis MO 63166-6550
Phone Number	800-256-8918
Fax Number	800-276-9901
Medications on Program	Androgel 1% Gel 2.5gm, 5gm (testosterone topical) Androgel 1% Pump (testosterone topical)
Application Forms	Abbott Labs Patient Assistance Program
Online Application	No online application available at this time Form: abbottgrowth-us.com/static/wma/pdf/1/6/1/1/3/ SolvayApplication0210.pdf
Eligibility Guidelines and Notes	The patient must have no prescription coverage for any medications and meet income guidelines that are not disclosed. Medical diagnosis necessary for this program is not specified. The patient must also be a US resident. If a patient did not enroll in Medicare Part D, then he may still be eligible for this program and should apply. If a patient has Part D and has been denied coverage, he may be considered by this program.
Application Process	With the patient's permission, anyone concerned can call for an application. The application can be either faxed or mailed out upon request. The completed application must be faxed or mailed from the doctor's office. The doctor or patient should call to check on status. The estimated timeline for acceptance is 7-10 business days. The medication is shipped within 2 business days.
Application Requirements	The doctor must fill out a section and sign the application. The patient must fill out a section, sign the application and attach proof of income.
Program Details	Up to a 90-day supply is sent to the doctor's office. The patient or doctor must contact the company for refills. Once a year a new application with financial documentation is needed.

Bibliography and Further Reading

Bhasin et al. **"Testosterone Therapy in Adult Men with Androgen Deficiency Syndromes: An Endocrine Society Clinical Practice Guideline".** The Journal of Clinical Endocrinology & Metabolism Vol. 91, No. 6 1995-2010. This are the American Association of Clinical Endocrinologists Medical Guidelines for Clinical Practice for the Evaluation and Treatment of Hypogonadism (You can read them at link 12 and 13 of www.aace.com/pub/guidelines/)

How to Order More Copies of This Book

This book is available at Amazon.com. For orders outside the United States, mail a bank-check or money order for US$30 (which includes shipping and handling) to: Nelson Vergel P.O.Box 667223. Houston, TX 77266

A Spanish translation will be available at the end of 2010 via Amazon. com titled "La Testosterona: Una Guia Para Hombres."

-APPENDIX C-

Compounding Pharmacies

Frequently Asked Questions About Compounding

(This comes from the International Academy of Compounding Pharmacists (IACP) www.iacprx.org)

What is pharmacy compounding?

Pharmacy compounding is the customized preparation of a medicine that is not otherwise commercially available. These medications are prescribed by a physician, veterinarian, or other prescribing practitioner, and compounded by a state-licensed pharmacist. A growing number of people and animals have unique health needs that off-the-shelf, one-size-fits-all prescription medicines cannot meet. For them, customized medications are the only way to better health.

Who are compounding pharmacists?

Pharmacy compounding is a centuries-old, well-regulated and common practice. Pharmacists are one of the most respected and trusted professionals in the United States. In a recent survey, pharmacists ranked second (only behind nurses) as the most trusted professionals in American society. Compounding has evolved into a specialty practice within the pharmacy community today. New applications to meet today's patient needs require additional education, equipment, and processes that not all pharmacies possess.

How are compounding pharmacies and pharmacists regulated? Should there be increased federal oversight?

All pharmacies and pharmacists are licensed and strictly regulated at the state level. Compounding is a core component of pharmacy and has always been regulated by state boards, which are constantly updating their standards and regulations. In addition, standards set by the United States Pharmacopeia (USP) are integrated into the practice of pharmacy compounding. The Pharmacy Compounding Accreditation Board (PCAB) has developed national standards to accredit pharmacies that perform a significant amount of compounding.

Does the FDA have the expertise and federal power to regulate compounding pharmacies? Why shouldn't compounded medications, especially the most commonly used combinations, have to go through FDA's established drug approval process?

The medical profession, including the practice of pharmacy, has always been regulated by the states. State boards of pharmacy are in the best position to inspect pharmacy operations, develop appropriate regulations, and respond to problems or violations. The FDA does have an important role to play in making sure that ingredients used in compounding are safe and are manufactured by the FDA-registered and inspected facilities, but there is no such thing as an "FDA-approved" pharmacy.

The FDA's drug approval process takes years and can cost hundreds of millions of dollars. Requiring this for individually personalized medications that fulfill an individual doctor's prescription is both impractical and contrary to the best interests of patients requiring immediate treatment.

What suppliers sell ingredients to compounding pharmacies? How are these suppliers regulated?

Just like big pharmaceutical manufacturing companies, compounding pharmacies get their ingredients for medications from the suppliers that are registered and inspected by the FDA. Foreign suppliers are FDA-registered facilities.

There are thousands of FDA-approved drugs on the market for just about any ailment. Why do we still need compounded medications?

Some valuable medications are only available by compounding. Restricting a doctor's access to compounded medications would be a serious mistake. Moreover, because of the economics of pharmaceutical manufacturing, FDA-approved drugs that serve a limited population are often discontinued by manufacturers. In most of these cases the only option left for doctors and their patients is to have a compounding pharmacist make the discontinued drug from scratch using pharmaceutical grade ingredients.

Are compounded medications safe? How does one know that the compounded medication they are taking is safe and effective?

Compounded medications are similar to the so-called off-label use of FDA-approved drugs. When the FDA approves a specific drug as safe and effective, this determination applies only to the specific disease or condition for which the drug was tested. But physicians and veterinarians often prescribe medications for treatments for which they have not been specifically approved. Medical professionals do this because, in their judgment, the treatment is in the best interest of the individual patient.

Similarly, medical professionals often prescribe compounded medications because they believe it is the best medical option for their patients. It is estimated that one fifth of all prescriptions written for FDA-approved drugs are for uses for which they were not specifically approved.

Some Compounding Pharmacies I Have Used:

This is a very small list of the compounding pharmacies that I have used. There are many more around the country, so I encourage you to Google "compounding pharmacy + your city" to find local ones. The ones listed here ship in the United States and require your physician to call in or fax a prescription. You should call them to compare prices and to provide your credit card and address information.APSMEDS.com (some of the best prices on testosterone gels, HCG, Clomid, etc)

GBTRX.com (also very reliable). They have a patient assistance program. The program is based on the Federal Poverty Guidelines. Discounts will range from 15% to 60%, depending on income level. The maximum level to qualify is 400% of the Federal Poverty Guidelines, or currently a gross income of $3,170.00 per month.

They can be reached at (866) 422-6770 or by email: garypetonke@gbtrx. com

GotoCompoundingShop.com (more expensive, but extremely reliable)
CollegePharmacy.com
Women's International Pharmacy (great for women's gels but they also sell men's products)
www.womensinternational.com/
Find a doctor who uses them
hwww.womensinternational.com/resources_referral.html
National Directory of Compounding Pharmacies:
www.angelfire.com/fl/endohystnhrt/pharmacy.html

-APPENDIX D-

PHYSICIANS WHO TREAT HYPOGONADISM

Most primary care doctors in the United States feel comfortable prescribing testosterone in 2010. After you find a potential doctor, ask some basic questions to determine their level of knowledge about testosterone. Some may feel insulted to be asked questions like these, but if they are it's probably not going to be a good match for you (of course, be nice and diplomatic when asking questions!)-

1. How many men does he/she treat for hypogonadism?
2. Does he/she offer HCG therapy, in addition to testosterone for testicular atrophy? (Many doctors do not know how to use HCG.)
3. Does he/she use Arimidex or tamoxifen to keep estrogen down in case of gynecomastia (enlarged breasts)?
4. Does he/she check for primary or secondary hypogonadism?
5. Does he/she allow patients to self-inject at home?
6. Does he/she work with any compounding pharmacies to access cheaper and customized hormonal products? (As mentioned previously, some doctors worry compounding pharmacies have poor quality control)
7. What does he/she think of AACE hypogonadism guidelines? (American Association of Clinical Endocrinologists Medical Guidelines for Clinical Practice for the Evaluation and Treatment of Hypogonadism). These guidelines are very clear and doctors who have *not* read them should not be prescribing testosterone and managing sexual dysfunction. You can read them at link 12 and 13 of www.aace.com/pub/guidelines/

Here are several resources that can help you if you need to search for one:

The Hormone Foundation

The Hormone Foundation, the public education affiliate of The Endocrine Society, is a leading source of hormone-related health information for the public, physicians, allied health professionals and the media. Their mission is to serve as a resource for the public by promoting the prevention, treatment and cure of hormone-related conditions through outreach and education.

The Hormone Foundation's physician referral directory is comprised of over 3,000 members of The Endocrine Society, the largest and most influential organization of endocrinologists in the world. The referral is updated weekly with physicians who are accepting new patients. To find a specialist near you, please use the search tools below. You can search by ZIP code, state/province, or area of specialty (e.g., diabetes, thyroid, etc.) within the United States and abroad.

www.endojournals.org/misc/patient_info.dtl

Life Extension Foundation, List of Innovative Doctors: www.lef.org/Health-Wellness/ InnovativeDoctors/

There is an AACE doctor search page at www.aace.com/memsearch. php

In theory they would use the AACE hypogonadism guidelines, but do not assume that all endocrinologists are testosterone friendly.

Find a doctor who uses the services of **Women's International Pharmacy**: www.womensinternational.com/resources_referral.html

College Pharmacy (Colorado Springs, CO)

http://www.collegepharmacy.com/
Click "Find a Health Care Provider." There is a form to fill out. Submit the form and they will e-mail a list of doctors nearest you who use their compounding services.

Medibolics.com, a HIV-related web site

Doctors in this list also treat people who are not HIV positive: www.medi-bolics.com/physic2.htm

Directory of "anti-aging" worldwide doctors

www.worldhealth.net/ pages/directory/

-APPENDIX E-

HOW TO JOIN TESTOSTERONE RESEARCH STUDIES

Those of you who want to help advance the understanding of testosterone use for different conditions can join research studies that are currently enrolling. I was amazed to see how many studies are out there!

Remember that some studies have placebo arms. Every study requires for you to read and sign a consent form that should clearly describe the risks and implications in joining the study. Make sure that the private investigator or research nurse overseeing the study explains things to you clearly.

Study to Determine the Long-Term Effects of Testosterone Replacement in Men (December 2009)

Unfortunately, there have been no controlled studies on the long-term use of testosterone replacement in men, even though many of us have been using it for over 20 years.

To answer questions about the long-term effect of testosterone replacement therapy in men the National Institute on Aging, part of the National Institutes of Health, announced the in November 2009 start of a large-scale clinical trial to evaluate the effect of testosterone therapy in older men. Led by researchers at the University of Pennsylvania School of Medicine and conducted at 12 sites across the nation, the testosterone trial will involve 800 men aged 65 years and older with low testosterone levels. The testosterone trial will include five separate studies. Men aged 65 years and older with low serum testosterone and at least one hypogonadal condition (anemia, decreased physical function, low vitality, impaired cognition, or reduced sexual function) will be randomly assigned to participate in a treatment group or a control group.

Treatment groups will be given a testosterone gel that is applied to the torso, abdomen, or upper arms. Control groups will receive a placebo gel. Serum testosterone will be measured monthly for the first three months and quarterly thereafter for up to one year. Participants will be tested on a wide range of measures to evaluate physical function, vitality, cognition, cardiovascular disease, and sexual function.

Volunteering for a trial can really help advance research. Men interested in finding out more about participating in the study should call one of the following institutions:

- University of California, Los Angeles; 310-222-5297
- University of California, San Diego; 877-219-6610
- Boston University; 617-414-2968
- University of Pittsburgh; 800-872-3653
- Albert Einstein College of Medicine, Bronx, N.Y.; 718-405-8271
- Baylor College of Medicine, Houston, Texas; 713-798-8343
- University of Minnesota, Minneapolis; 612-625-4449
- Yale University, New Haven, Conn.; 203-737-5672
- University of Alabama at Birmingham; 205-934-2294
- *VA* Puget Sound Health Care System and University of Washington School of Medicine, Seattle; 206-768-5408
- Northwestern University, Evanston, Ill.; 877-300-3065
- University of Florida, Gainesville; 866-386-7730, 352-273-5919

Other Studies:

This is a list obtained from clinicaltrials.gov in summer of 2010 (visit the respective link to find out more about every study. This is a great way to not only have access to therapy, but also to have great monitoring and to serve for the better of humanity):

Title: Exogenous Testosterone Plus Dutasteride for the Treatment of Castrate Metastatic Prostate Cancer

Recruitment:	Recruiting
Conditions:	Prostate Cancer|Castration-resistant, Metastatic
Interventions:	Other: testosterone (AndroGel®) with the 5α-reductase inhibitor dutasteride
URL:	http://ClinicalTrials.gov/show/NCT00853697

Title: Anabolic and Inflammatory Responses to Short-Term Testosterone Administration in Older Men

Recruitment:	Recruiting
Conditions:	Sarcopenia
Interventions:	Drug: Testosterone injection|Drug: Testosterone gel
URL:	http://ClinicalTrials.gov/show/NCT00957801

Title: Testosterone for Penile Rehab After Radical Prostatectomy

Recruitment:	Recruiting
Conditions:	Low Testosterone Levels|Erectile Dysfunction
Interventions:	Drug: Testim® + Viagra®|Drug: Placebo Testim® + Viagra®
URL:	http://ClinicalTrials.gov/show/NCT00848497

Title: Use of Nebido® to Assess Tolerability and Treatment Outcomes in Daily Clinical Practice

Recruitment:	Recruiting
Conditions:	Male|Hypogonadism
Interventions:	Drug: Testosterone Undecanoate (Nebido, BAY86-5037)
URL:	http://ClinicalTrials.gov/show/NCT00410306

Title: Pharmacokinetic and Comparative Bioavailability Study of Testosterone Absorption after Administration of Testosterone Gel 1.62% to the Upper Arms/Shoulders Using an Application Site Rotation or a Combination of Application Sites in Hypogonadal Males

Recruitment:	Recruiting
Conditions:	Hypogonadism
Interventions:	Drug: Testosterone Gel 1.62%|Drug: Testosterone Gel 1.62%
URL:	http://ClinicalTrials.gov/show/NCT01133548

Title: Effect of Testosterone on Endothelial Function and Microcirculation in Type 2 Diabetic Patients With Hypogonadism

Recruitment:	Not yet recruiting
Conditions:	Type 2 Diabetes|Hypogonadism
Interventions:	Drug: Testosterone
URL:	http://ClinicalTrials.gov/show/NCT01084369

Title: An Open-Label Study of Serum Testosterone Levels in Non-dosed Females After Secondary Exposure to Testosterone Gel 1.62% Applied to the Upper Arms and Shoulders and Use of a T-shirt Barrier

Recruitment:	Recruiting
Conditions:	Pharmacokinetics
Interventions:	Drug: Testosterone Gel 1.62%
URL:	http://ClinicalTrials.gov/show/NCT01130298

Title: Testosterone Replacement for Fatigue in Male Hypogonadic Advanced Cancer Patients

Recruitment:	Recruiting
Conditions:	Advanced Cancer
Interventions:	Drug: Testosterone|Drug: Placebo
URL:	http://ClinicalTrials.gov/show/NCT00965341

Title: Effect of Testosterone in Men With Erectile Dysfunction

Recruitment:	Recruiting
Conditions:	Erectile Dysfunction|Testosterone Deficiency|Diabetes
Interventions:	Drug: Sildenafil citrate (open label)|Drug: Testosterone gel 1% (active or placebo)|Drug: Topical testosterone gel 1%
URL:	http://ClinicalTrials.gov/show/NCT00512707

Title: Influence of Administration Route of Testosterone on Male Fertility

Recruitment:	Not yet recruiting
Conditions:	Hypogonadism
Interventions:	Drug: MPP10, testosterone|Drug: Testosterone
URL:	http://ClinicalTrials.gov/show/NCT00705796

Title: NASOBOL in Hypogonadal Men in Comparison to Testosterone Levels in Normal Healthy Male Volunteers

Recruitment:	Recruiting
Conditions:	Hypogonadism
Interventions:	Drug: testosterone|Other: No treatment
URL:	http://ClinicalTrials.gov/show/NCT00647868

Title: Effect of Testosterone Gel Replacement on Fat Mass in Males With Low Testosterone Levels and Diabetes

Recruitment:	Not yet recruiting
Conditions:	Hypogonadism|Diabetes
Interventions:	Drug: Testosterone gel|Drug: placebo
URL:	http://ClinicalTrials.gov/show/NCT00440440

Title: The Testosterone Trial

Recruitment:	Recruiting
Conditions:	Andropause
Interventions:	Drug: AndroGel® (testosterone gel)
URL:	http://ClinicalTrials.gov/show/NCT00799617

Title: Vaginal Testosterone Cream vs ESTRING for Vaginal Dryness or Decreased Libido in Early Stage Breast Cancer Patients

Recruitment:	Recruiting
Conditions:	Sexual Dysfunction, Physiological
Interventions:	Drug: Testosterone Cream|Drug: Estring
URL:	http://ClinicalTrials.gov/show/NCT00698035

Title: Effect of Testosterone Therapy in Men With Alzheimer's Disease and Low Testosterone

Recruitment:	Recruiting
Conditions:	Alzheimer's Disease|Hypogonadism
Interventions:	Drug: AndroGel (Solvay Pharmaceuticals)
URL:	http://ClinicalTrials.gov/show/NCT00392912

Title: 5-Alpha Reductase and Anabolic Effects of Testosterone

Recruitment:	Recruiting
Conditions:	Male Hypogonadism|Muscle Atrophy|Prostate Enlargement| Sarcopenia

Interventions: Drug: Testosterone Enanthate|Behavioral: Collection
                   of 3-day food logs with counseling of subjects|Drug:
                   Finasteride|Behavioral: Collection of 3-day food
                   logs with counseling of subjects|Drug: Testosterone
                   Enanthate|Drug: Finasteride|Behavioral: Collection of
                   3-day food logs with counseling of subjects
URL: http://ClinicalTrials.gov/show/NCT00475501

Title: Effects of Testosterone Replacement on Pain Sensitivity and Pain Perception
Recruitment: Recruiting
Study Results: No Results Available
Conditions: Pain|Hypogonadism
Interventions: Drug: Androgel (testosterone gel)|Other: Placebo
URL: http://ClinicalTrials.gov/show/NCT00351819

Title: Testosterone Gel Applied to Women With Pituitary Gland Problems
Recruitment: Recruiting
Conditions: Panhypopituitarism
Interventions: Drug: Transdermal Testosterone gel
URL: http://ClinicalTrials.gov/show/NCT00144391

Title: Testosterone Therapy in Men With Low Testosterone Levels and Metabolic Syndrome or Early Stages of Type 2 Diabetes
Recruitment: Recruiting
Conditions: Metabolic Syndrome
Interventions: Drug: Transdermal testosterone therapy|Drug: Placebo
URL: http://ClinicalTrials.gov/show/NCT00479609

Title: Effect of Testosterone Replacement on Insulin Resistance
Recruitment: Recruiting
Conditions: Metabolic Syndrome|Hypogonadism
Interventions: Radiation: Testosterone gel|Drug: Placebo for testos-
                   terone gel
URL: http://ClinicalTrials.gov/show/NCT00487734

Title: Effect of Androgel on Type 2 Diabetic Males With Hypogonadism

Recruitment:	Recruiting
Conditions:	Diabetes Mellitus Type 2
Interventions:	Drug: Testosterone(AndroGel)
URL:	http://ClinicalTrials.gov/show/NCT00350701

Title: TEAM: Testosterone Supplementation and Exercise in Elderly Men

Recruitment:	Recruiting
Conditions:	Healthy
Interventions:	Drug: Testosterone Gel|Behavioral: Exercise - Progressive Resistance Training (PRT)|Drug: Placebo Gel
URL:	http://ClinicalTrials.gov/show/NCT00112151

Title: Dose Titration Investigation of the Pharmacokinetics of Testosterone Transdermal Systems in Hypogonadal Men

Recruitment:	Recruiting
Conditions:	Hypogonadism
Interventions:	Drug: Testerone Transdermal System
URL:	http://ClinicalTrials.gov/show/NCT01104246

Title: Testosterone for Peripheral Vascular Disease

Recruitment:	Recruiting
Conditions:	Hypogonadism|Peripheral Vascular Disease|Type 2 Diabetes
Interventions:	Drug: Testosterone|Drug: 0.9% saline
URL:	http://ClinicalTrials.gov/show/NCT00504712

Title: A Pilot Study of Parenteral Testosterone and Oral Etoposide as Therapy for Men With Castration Resistant Prostate Cancer

Recruitment:	Recruiting
Conditions:	Prostate Cancer
Interventions:	Drug: Testosterone|Drug: Etoposide
URL:	http://ClinicalTrials.gov/show/NCT01084759

Title: Efficacy and Tolerability of an Intra-Nasal Testosterone Product

Recruitment: Recruiting
Conditions: Hypogonadism
Interventions: Drug: Nasobol® (Itra-nasal Testosterone)|Drug:
                Androderm® (Positive Control)
URL: http://ClinicalTrials.gov/show/NCT00975650

Title: Testosterone Replacement in Men With Diabetes and Obesity

Recruitment: Recruiting
Conditions: Hypogonadism
Interventions: Drug: testosterone|Drug: placebo
URL: http://ClinicalTrials.gov/show/NCT01127659

Title: NEBIDO in Symptomatic Late Onset Hypogonadism (SLOH)

Recruitment: Not yet recruiting
Conditions: Hypogonadism
Interventions: Drug: Testosterone Undeconate (Nebido, BAY86-
                5037)|Drug: Placebo
URL: http://ClinicalTrials.gov/show/NCT01092858

Title: Baseline Sexual Function, Cognitive Function, Body Composition and Muscle Parameters and Pharmacokinetics of Transdermal Testosterone Gel in Women With Hypopituitarism

Recruitment: Recruiting
Conditions: Panhypopituitarism
Interventions: Drug: Transdermal Testosterone Gel
URL: http://ClinicalTrials.gov/show/NCT00144404

Title:Effect of Increasing Testosterone on Insulin Sensitivity in Men With the Metabolic Syndrome

Recruitment: Recruiting
Conditions: Metabolic Syndrome
Interventions: Drug: Zoladex|Drug: AndroGel|Drug: Arimidex
URL: http://ClinicalTrials.gov/show/NCT00438321

Title: Testosterone Replacement in Men With Non-Metastatic Castrate Resistant Prostate Cancer

Recruitment: Recruiting
Conditions: Prostate Cancer
Interventions: Drug: AndroGel|Drug: placebo
URL: http://ClinicalTrials.gov/show/NCT00515112

Title: The Effect of IM Testosterone Undecanoate on Biochemical and Anthropometric Characteristics of Metabolic Syndrome in Hypogonadal Men

Recruitment: Recruiting
Conditions: Metabolic Syndrome|Hypogonadism
Interventions: Drug: Nebido (testosterone undecanoate)|Drug: Placebo
URL: http://ClinicalTrials.gov/show/NCT00696748

Title: The Therapy of Nebido as Mono or in Combination With PDE-5 Inhibitors in Hypogonadal Patients With Erectile Dysfunction

Recruitment: Recruiting
Conditions: Hypogonadism|Erectile Dysfunction
Interventions: Drug: Testosterone undecanoate
URL: http://ClinicalTrials.gov/show/NCT00421460

Title: Transdermal Testosterone Gel/Effect on Erection Quality as Measured by DIR

Recruitment: Recruiting
Conditions: Hypogonadism
Interventions: Drug: AndroGel (Transdermal Testosterone Gel)
URL: http://ClinicalTrials.gov/show/NCT00425568

Title: The Effect of 5-Alpha Reductase on Testosterone in Men

Recruitment: Recruiting
Conditions: Sex Disorders
Interventions: Drug: testosterone enanthate|Drug: duastride
URL: http://ClinicalTrials.gov/show/NCT00070733

Title: Treatment of Erectile Dysfunction in Hypogonadal Men With Testosterone Undecanoate

Recruitment:	Recruiting
Conditions:	Erectile Dysfunction|Hypogonadotrophic Males
Interventions:	Drug: Testosterone Undecanoate and/or PDE-5
URL:	http://ClinicalTrials.gov/show/NCT00555087

Title: Analgesic Efficacy of Testosterone Replacement in Hypogonadal Opioid-Treated Chronic Pain Patients: A Pilot Study.

Recruitment:	Recruiting
Conditions:	Pain|Hypogonadism
Interventions:	Drug: Testosterone Gel
URL:	http://ClinicalTrials.gov/show/NCT00398034

Title:Anabolic Therapies: New Hope for Treating Secondary Disabilities of SCI

Recruitment:	Recruiting
Conditions:	Hypogonadism|Spinal Cord Injury
Interventions:	Drug: Testosterone Replacement Therapy Patch 5mg daily
URL:	http://ClinicalTrials.gov/show/NCT00266864

Title:Does Testosterone Improve Function in Hypogonadal Older Men

Recruitment:	Recruiting
Conditions:	Hypogonadism
Interventions:	Drug: Testosterone
URL:	http://ClinicalTrials.gov/show/NCT00304213

Title:The Effect of Testosterone Replacement on Bone Mineral Density in Boys and Men With Anorexia Nervosa

Recruitment:	Recruiting
Conditions:	Bone Metabolism
Interventions:	Drug: testosterone cypionate|Other: Bone monitoring
URL:	http://ClinicalTrials.gov/show/NCT00853502

Title: Effects of Testosterone in Women With Depression

Recruitment:	Recruiting
Conditions:	Depression

Interventions: Drug: Testosterone
URL: http://ClinicalTrials.gov/show/NCT00676676

Title: Reandron in Diabetic Men Witn Low Testosterone Level
Recruitment: Recruiting
Conditions: Type 2 Diabetes|Hypogonadism
Interventions: Drug: Reandron 1000|Drug: placebo
URL: http://ClinicalTrials.gov/show/NCT00613782

Title: Outcomes of Mechanically Ventilated Patients With Low Serum Testosterone
Recruitment: Recruiting
Study Results: No Results Available
Conditions: Acute Respiratory Failure
Interventions:
URL: http://ClinicalTrials.gov/show/NCT00797433

Title: Testosterone Therapy on Angina Threshold and Atheroma in Patients With Chronic Stable Angina
Recruitment: Recruiting
Conditions: Angina Pectoris
Interventions: Drug: Nebido
URL: http://ClinicalTrials.gov/show/NCT00131183

Title: Hormone and Information Processing Study
Recruitment: Recruiting
Conditions: Mild Cognitive Impairment|Alzheimer's Disease
Interventions: Drug: testosterone gel|Drug: placebo gel
URL: http://ClinicalTrials.gov/show/NCT00539305

Title: Efficacy Study for Use of Dutasteride (Avodart) With Testosterone Replacement
Recruitment: Recruiting
Conditions: Hypogonadism
Interventions: Drug: dutasteride|Drug: placebo
URL: http://ClinicalTrials.gov/show/NCT00752869

Title: Testosterone Replacement in Middle-Aged Hypogonadal Men With Dysthymia: Parallel Group, Double Blind Randomized Trial

Recruitment:	Recruiting
Conditions:	Dysthymic Disorder
Interventions:	Drug: Testoviron
URL:	http://ClinicalTrials.gov/show/NCT00260390

Title:Decreased Testosterone Levels in Men Over 65

Recruitment:	Recruiting
Conditions:	Aging|Hypogonadism|Andropause
Interventions:	Drug: Anastrozole|Drug: Testosterone Gel|Drug: Placebo tablet|Drug: Placebo gel|Dietary Supplement: Calcium Cardone 500mg with vitamin D 400 IU
URL:	http://ClinicalTrials.gov/show/NCT00104572

Title:Testosterone Replacement Therapy in Advanced Chronic Kidney Disease

Recruitment:	Recruiting
Study Results:	No Results Available
Conditions:	Kidney Failure|Kidney Diseases
Interventions:	Drug: Testim (1% testosterone gel)
URL:	http://ClinicalTrials.gov/show/NCT00645658

Title:The Cardiac Benefit of Testosterone Replacement in Men With Low Testosterone Levels With Coronary Artery Disease After Successful Intervention of the Blockage or Narrowed Heart Artery

Recruitment:	Recruiting
Conditions:	Coronary Artery Disease
Interventions:	Drug: AndroGel 5 Grams
URL:	http://ClinicalTrials.gov/show/NCT00413244

Title:Dose-Response of Gonadal Steroids and Bone Turnover in Men

Recruitment:	Recruiting
Conditions:	Healthy Volunteers
Interventions:	Drug: testosterone|Drug: goserelin acetate|Drug: anastrazole
URL:	http://ClinicalTrials.gov/show/NCT00114114

Title: Effect of Androgel on Atherogenesis, Inflammation, Cardiovascular Risk Factors And Adiposity in Type 2 Diabetic Males With Hypogonadotrophic Hypogonadism

Recruitment:	Not yet recruiting
Conditions:	Type 2 Diabetic Male With Hypogonadotrophic Hypogonadism.
Interventions:	Drug: Androgel
URL:	http://ClinicalTrials.gov/show/NCT00467987

Title: Hormonal Factors in the Treatment of Anorexia Nervosa

Recruitment:	Recruiting
Conditions:	Anorexia Nervosa|Eating Disorder|Anxiety|Depression
Interventions:	Drug: Testosterone|Drug: Placebo
URL:	http://ClinicalTrials.gov/show/NCT01121211

Title: Investigator Initiated Study of the Effects of Androgen Therapy on Carbohydrate and Lipid Metabolism In Elderly Men

Recruitment:	Recruiting
Conditions:	Aging|Obesity|Insulin Resistance|Hypogonadism
Interventions:	Drug: Topical testosterone (Androgel) 10 g/day
URL:	http://ClinicalTrials.gov/show/NCT00365794

Title: Phase II Randomized Study of Physiologic Testosterone Replacement in Premenopausal, HIV-Positive Women

Recruitment:	Recruiting
Conditions:	HIV Infections|Cachexia
Interventions:	Drug: testosterone
URL:	http://ClinicalTrials.gov/show/NCT00004400

Title: Amino Acid Supplement and/or Testosterone in Treating Cachexia in Patients With Advanced or Recurrent Cervical Cancer

Recruitment:	Recruiting
Conditions:	Cachexia|Cervical Cancer
Interventions:	Dietary Supplement: leucine-enhanced essential amino acid dietary supplement|Drug: therapeutic testosterone|Other: placebo
URL:	http://ClinicalTrials.gov/show/NCT00878995

Title: Deslorelin Combined With Low-Dose Add-Back Estradiol and Testosterone in Preventing Breast Cancer in Premenopausal Women Who Are at High Risk for This Disease

Recruitment: Recruiting

Conditions: brca1 Mutation Carrier|brca2 Mutation Carrier|Breast Cancer

Interventions: Biological: therapeutic estradiol|Drug: deslorelin|Drug: therapeutic testosterone

URL: http://ClinicalTrials.gov/show/NCT00080756

Title: Effect of High Testosterone on Sleep-associated Slowing of Follicular Luteinizing Hormone (LH) Frequency in Polycystic Ovary Syndrome

Recruitment: Recruiting

Conditions: Polycystic Ovary Syndrome

Interventions: Drug: Flutamide|Drug: Placebo

URL: http://ClinicalTrials.gov/show/NCT00930228

Title: Metabolic Effects of Androgenicity in Aging Men and Women

Recruitment: Recruiting

Conditions: Aging|Insulin Resistance

Interventions: Drug: Testosterone|Drug: Estrogen

URL: http://ClinicalTrials.gov/show/NCT00680797

Title:Sleep-wake Changes of Luteinizing Hormone Frequency in Pubertal Girls With and Without High Testosterone

Recruitment: Recruiting

Conditions: Hyperandrogenism

Interventions:

URL: http://ClinicalTrials.gov/show/NCT00930007

Title:Safety and Efficacy of LibiGel® for the Treatment of Hypoactive Sexual Desire Disorder in Surgically Menopausal Women

Recruitment: Recruiting

Conditions: Hypoactive Sexual Desire Disorder

Interventions: Drug: testosterone gel|Drug: placebo gel

URL: http://ClinicalTrials.gov/show/NCT00613002

Title: Safety and Efficacy of LibiGel® for Treatment of Hypoactive Sexual Desire Disorder in Postmenopausal Women

Recruitment:	Recruiting
Conditions:	Hypoactive Sexual Desire Disorder
Interventions:	Drug: testosterone gel|Drug: placebo gel
URL:	http://ClinicalTrials.gov/show/NCT00612742

Title: Sexual Dysfunction And Hypotestosteronemia In Patients With Obstructive Sleep Apnea Syndrome And Its Effects With CPAP Therapy

Recruitment:	Recruiting
Conditions:	Obstructive Sleep Apnea Syndrome (OSAS)|Sleep Apnea|Hypotestosteronemia
Interventions:	
URL:	http://ClinicalTrials.gov/show/NCT00832065

Title: Surveillance Study of Women Taking Intrinsa®

Recruitment:	Recruiting
Study Results:	No Results Available
Conditions:	Ovariectomy|Hysterectomy|Hypoactive Sexual Desire Disorder
Interventions:	
URL:	http://ClinicalTrials.gov/show/NCT00551785

Title: Safety and Efficacy of LibiGel® for Treatment of Hypoactive Sexual Desire Disorder in Surgically Menopausal Women

Recruitment:	Recruiting
Conditions:	Hypoactive Sexual Desire Disorder
Interventions:	Drug: testosterone gel|Drug: placebo gel
URL:	http://ClinicalTrials.gov/show/NCT00657501
Interventions:	Procedure: Stable Isotope Infusion Study|Procedure: Collection of blood and tissues|Procedure: Radiology testing: DEXA, K+ counter, ultrasound, MRI|Drug: Humatrope|Drug: Ketoconazole|Drug: Oxandrolone|Drug: Propranolol|Drug: Oxandrolone and propranolol combined|Drug: Humatrope and propranolol combined|Drug: Placebo|Behavioral:

Exercise--Hospital supervised intensive exercise
program|Behavioral: Home exercise program
URL: http://ClinicalTrials.gov/show/NCT00675714

Title: Registry of Hypogonadism in Men
Recruitment: Recruiting
Conditions: Male   Hypogonadism|Androgen   Deficiency|
                 Testosterone Deficiency
Interventions: Other: Standard of Care
URL: http://ClinicalTrials.gov/show/NCT00858650

Title: Sex Steroids, Sleep, and Metabolic Dysfunction in Women
Recruitment: Recruiting
Study Results: No Results Available
Conditions: Polycystic   Ovary   Syndrome|Obstructive   Sleep
                 Apnea|Obesity
Interventions: Drug: Progesterone|Drug: testosterone|Drug:
                 glucocorticoid|Device: continuous positive airway
                 pressure
URL: http://ClinicalTrials.gov/show/NCT00805207

Title: Adolescent Cooking and Eating Study
Recruitment: Not yet recruiting
Conditions: Polycystic Ovary Syndrome
Interventions: Behavioral: Nutrition Education, Dietary Counseling,
                 and Cooking
URL: http://ClinicalTrials.gov/show/NCT01079845

Title: Studying the Effects of 7 Days of Gonadotropin Releasing Hormone (GnRH) Treatment in Men With Hypogonadism
Recruitment: Recruiting
Conditions: Kallmann   Syndrome|Idiopathic   Hypogonadotropic
                 Hypogonadism
Interventions: Drug: gonadotropin releasing hormone (GnRH)
URL: http://ClinicalTrials.gov/show/NCT00493961

Title: Follicle Stimulating Hormone (FSH) to Improve Testicular Development in Men With Hypogonadism

Recruitment:	Recruiting
Conditions:	Hypogonadism|Kallmann Syndrome
Interventions:	Procedure: Testicular biopsy|Drug: gonadotropin releasing hormone (GnRH)|Drug: follicle stimulating hormone (FSH)
URL:	http://ClinicalTrials.gov/show/NCT00064987

Title: Prevalence of Hypogonadism in Male Cancer Patients

Recruitment:	Recruiting
Conditions:	Cancer|Hypogonadism
Interventions:	
URL:	http://ClinicalTrials.gov/show/NCT00472940

-APPENDIX F-

Testosterone Physician's Desk Reference Package Inserts for an Injectable and a Gel

This package insert is included in all testosterone replacement products available in the market. This one specifically mentions testosterone enanthate, but this information applies to all testosterones. Be aware that some of the liver-related side effects mentioned have been linked mostly with oral formulations that are no longer used.

DESCRIPTION

DELATESTRYL® (Testosterone Enanthate Injection, USP) provides testosterone enanthate, a derivative of the primary endogenous androgen testosterone, for intramuscular administration. In their active form, androgens have a 17-beta-hydroxy group. Esterification of the 17-beta-hydroxy group increases the duration of action of testosterone; hydrolysis to free testosterone occurs *in vivo*. Each milliliter of sterile, colorless to pale yellow solution provides 200 mg of testosterone enanthate in sesame oil with 5 mg of chlorobutanol (chloral derivative) as a preservative.

Testosterone enanthate is designated chemically as androst-4-en-3-one, l7-[(l-oxoheptyl)-oxy]-, (17/?)-. Structural formula:

$$C_{26}H_{40}O_3$$
$$MW: 400.6$$

CLINICAL PHARMACOLOGY

Endogenous androgens are responsible for the normal growth and development of male sex organs and for maintenance of secondary sex characteristics. These effects include growth and maturation of prostate, seminal vesicles, penis, and scrotum; development of male hair distribution, such as beard, pubic, chest, and axillary hair; laryngeal enlargement; vocal chord thickening; alterations in body musculature; and fat distribution.

Androgens also cause retention of nitrogen, sodium, potassium, and phosphorus, and decrease urinary excretion of calcium. Androgens have been reported to increase protein anabolism and decrease protein catabolism. Nitrogen balance is improved only when there is sufficient intake of calories and protein.

Androgens are responsible for the growth spurt of adolescence and for the eventual termination of linear growth which is brought about by the fusion of epiphyseal growth centers. In children, exogenous androgens accelerate linear growth rates but may cause a disproportionate advancement in bone maturation. Use of androgens over long periods may result in the fusion of epiphyseal growth centers and termination of the growth process. Androgens have been reported to stimulate the production of red blood cells by enhancing the production of erythropoietic stimulating factor.

During exogenous administration of androgens, endogenous testosterone release is inhibited through feedback inhibition of pituitary LH. At large doses of exogenous androgens, spermatogenesis may also be suppressed through feedback inhibition of pituitary FSH.

There is a lack of substantial evidence that androgens are effective in fractures, surgery, convalescence, and functional uterine bleeding.

PHARMACOKINETICS

Testosterone esters are less polar than free testosterone do. Testosterone esters in oil-injected intramuscularly are absorbed slowly from the lipid phase; thus testosterone enanthate can be given at intervals of 2 to 4 weeks.

Testosterone in plasma is 98 percent bound to a specific testosterone-estradiol binding globulin, and about 2 percent is free. Generally, the amount of this sex-hormone binding globulin (SHBG) in the plasma will determine the distribution of testosterone between free and bound forms, and the free testosterone concentration will determine its half-life.

About 90 percent of a dose of testosterone is excreted in the urine as glucuronic and sulfuric acid conjugates of testosterone and its metabolites; about 6 percent of a dose is excreted in the feces, mostly in the unconjugated form. Inactivation of testosterone occurs primarily in the liver. Testosterone is metabolized to various 17-keto steroids through two different pathways. There are considerable variations of the half-life of testosterone as reported in the literature, ranging from 10 to 100 minutes.

In responsive tissues, the activity of testosterone appears to depend on reduction of DHT, which binds to cytosol receptor proteins. The steroid-receptor complex is transported to the nucleus where it initiates transcription events and cellular changes related to androgen action.

INDICATIONS AND USAGE

Males

DELATESTRYL® (Testosterone Enanthate Injection, USP) is indicated for replacement therapy in conditions associated with a deficiency or absence of endogenous testosterone.

Primary hypogonadism (congenital or acquired)—Testicular failure due to cryptorchidism, bilateral torsion, orchitis, vanishing testis syndrome, or orchidectomy.

Hypogonadotropic hypogonadism (congenital or acquired)—Idiopathic gonadotropin or luteinizing hormone-releasing hormone (LHRH) deficiency, or pituitary-hypothalamic injury from tumors, trauma, or radiation. (Appropriate adrenal cortical and thyroid hormone replacement therapy are still necessary, however, and are actually of primary importance.)

If the above conditions occur before puberty, androgen replacement therapy will be needed during the adolescent years for development of secondary sexual characteristics. Prolonged androgen treatment will be required to maintain sexual characteristics in these and other males who develop testosterone deficiency after puberty.Delayed puberty—DELATESTRYL® (Testosterone Enanthate Injection, USP) may be used to stimulate puberty in carefully selected males with clearly delayed puberty. These patients usually have a familial pattern of delayed puberty that is not secondary to a pathological disorder; puberty is expected to occur spontaneously at a relatively late date. Brief treatment with conservative doses may occasionally be justified in these patients if they do not respond to psychological support. The potential adverse effect on bone maturation should be discussed with the patient and parents before androgen administration. An X-ray of the hand and wrist to determine bone age should be done every 6 months to assess the effect of treatment on epiphyseal centers (see section WARNINGS).

Females

Metastatic mammary cancer—DELATESTRYL® (Testosterone Enanthate Injection, USP) may be used secondarily in women with advancing inoperable metastatic (skeletal) mammary cancer who are 1 to 5 years postmenopausal. Primary goals of therapy in these women include ablation of the ovaries. Other methods of counteracting estrogen activity are adrenalectomy, hypophysectomy, and/or antiestrogen therapy. This treatment has also been used in premenopausal women with breast cancer who have benefited from oophorectomy and are considered to have a hormone-responsive tumor. Judgment concerning androgen therapy should be made by an oncologist with expertise in this field.

Contraindications

Androgens are contraindicated in men with carcinomas of the breast or with known or suspected carcinomas of the prostate and in women who are or may become pregnant. When administered in pregnant women, androgens cause virilization of the external genitalia of the female fetus. This virilization includes clitoromegaly, abnormal vaginal development, and fusion of genital folds to form a scrotal-like structure. The degree of masculinization is related to the amount of drug given and the age of the fetus and is most likely to occur in the female fetus when the drugs are given in the first trimester. If the patient becomes pregnant while taking androgens, she should be apprised of the potential hazard to the fetus.

This preparation is also contraindicated in patients with a history of hyper-sensitivity to any of its components.

WARNINGS

In patients with breast cancer and in immobilized patients, androgen therapy may cause hypercalcemia by stimulating osteolysis. In patients with cancer, hypercalcemia may indicate progression of bony metastasis. If hypercal-cemia occurs, the drug should be discontinued and appropriate measures instituted.

Prolonged use of high doses of androgens has been associated with the development of peliosis hepatis and hepatic neoplasms including hepato-cellular carcinoma (see section PRECAUTIONS, Carcinogenesis). Peliosis hepatis can be a life-threatening or fatal complication.

If cholestatic hepatitis with jaundice appears or if liver function tests become abnormal, the androgen should be discontinued and the etiology should be determined. Drug-induced jaundice is reversible when the medication is discontinued.

Geriatric patients treated with androgens may be at an increased risk for the development of prostatic hypertrophy and prostatic carcinoma.

Due to sodium and water retention, edema with or without congestive heart failure may be a serious complication in patients with preexisting cardiac, renal, or hepatic disease. In addition to discontinuation of the drug, diuretic therapy may be required. If the administration of testosterone enanthate is restarted, a lower dose should be used.

Gynecomastia frequently develops and occasionally persists in patients being treated for hypogonadism.

Androgen therapy should be used cautiously in healthy males with delayed puberty. The effect on bone maturation should be monitored by assessing bone age of the wrist and hand every 6 months. In children, androgen treatment may accelerate bone maturation without producing compensatory gain in linear growth. This adverse effect may result in compromised adult stature. The younger the child, the greater the risk of compromising final mature height.

PRECAUTIONS

General

Women should be observed for signs of virilization (deepening of the voice, hirsutism, acne, clitoromegaly, and menstrual irregularities). Discontinuation of drug therapy at the time of evidence of mild virilism is necessary to prevent irreversible virilization. Such virilization is usual following androgen use at high doses and is not prevented by concomitant use of estrogens. A decision may be made by the patient and the physician that some virilization will be tolerated during treatment for breast carcinoma.

Because androgens may alter serum cholesterol concentration, caution should be exercised when administering these drugs to patients with a history of myocardial infarction or coronary artery disease. Serial determinations of serum cholesterol should be made and therapy adjusted accordingly. A causal relationship between myocardial infarction and hypercholesterolemia has not been established.

Information for Patients

Male adolescent patients receiving androgens for delayed puberty should have bone development checked every 6 months.

The physician should instruct patients to report any of the following side effects of androgens:

Adult or adolescent males—too frequent or persistent erections of the penis. Women—hoarseness, acne, changes in menstrual periods, or more facial hair. All patients—any nausea, vomiting, changes in skin color, or ankle swelling.

Geriatric Use

Clinical studies of DELATESTRYL did not include sufficient numbers of subjects, aged 65 years and older, to determine whether they respond differently from younger subjects. Testosterone replacement therapy is not indicated in geriatric patients who have age-related hypogonadism only ("andropause"), because there is insufficient safety and efficacy information to support such use. Current studies do not assess whether testosterone use increases the risks of prostate cancer, prostate hyperplasia, and cardiovascular disease in the geriatric population.

Intramuscular Administration

When properly given, injections of DELATESTRYL are well tolerated. Care should be taken to slowly inject the preparation deeply into the gluteal muscle, being sure to follow the usual precautions for intramuscular administration, such as the avoidance of intravascular injection. There have been rare postmarketing reports of transient reactions involving urge to cough, coughing fits, and respiratory distress immediately after the injection of DELATESTRYL, an oil-based depot preparation (see section 13, DOSAGE AND ADMINISTRATION).

Laboratory Tests

Women with disseminated breast carcinoma should have frequent determination of urine and serum calcium levels during the course of androgen therapy (see section WARNINGS).

Periodic (every 6 months) X-ray examinations of bone age should be made during treatment of pre-pubertal males to determine the rate of bone maturation and the effects of androgen therapy on the epiphyseal centers.

Hemoglobin and hematocrit should be checked periodically for polycythemia in patients who are receiving high doses of androgens.

Drug Interactions

When administered concurrently, the following drugs may interact with androgens.

Anticoagulants, oral – C-17 substituted derivatives of testosterone, such as methandrostenolone, have been reported to decrease the anticoagulant requirement. Patients receiving oral anticoagulant therapy require close monitoring especially when androgens are started or stopped.

Antidiabetic drugs and insulin—In diabetic patients, the metabolic effects of androgens may decrease blood glucose and insulin requirements.

ACTH and corticosteroids—Enhanced tendency toward edema. Exercise caution while administering these drugs together, especially in patients with hepatic or cardiac disease.

Oxyphenbutazone – Elevated serum levels of oxyphenbutazone may result.

Drug/Laboratory Test Interferences
Androgens may decrease levels of thyroxine-binding globulin, resulting in decreased total T4 serum levels and increased resin uptake of T3 and T4. Free thyroid hormone levels remain unchanged; however, there is no clinical evidence of thyroid dysfunction.

Carcinogenesis
Testosterone has been tested by subcutaneous injection and implantation in mice and rats. The implant induced cervical-uterine tumors in mice, which metastasized in some cases. There is suggestive evidence that injection of testosterone into some strains of female mice increases their susceptibility to hepatoma. Testosterone is also known to increase the number of tumors and decrease the degree of differentiation of chemically induced carcinomas of the liver in rats.

There are rare reports of hepatocellular carcinoma in patients receiving long-term therapy with androgens in high doses. Withdrawal of the drugs did not lead to regression of tumors in all cases.

Geriatric patients treated with androgens may be at an increased risk for the development of prostatic hypertrophy and prostatic carcinoma.

Pregnancy: Teratogenic Effects
Category X (see section CONTRAINDICATIONS).

Nursing Mothers
It is not known whether androgens are excreted in human milk. Because many drugs are excreted in human milk and because of the potential for serious adverse reactions in nursing infants from androgens, a decision should be made whether to discontinue nursing or to discontinue the drug, taking into account the importance of the drug to the mother.

Pediatric Use
Androgen therapy should be used very cautiously in pediatric patients and only by specialists who are aware of the adverse effects on bone maturation. Skeletal maturation must be monitored every 6 months by an X-ray of the hand and wrist (see section INDICATIONS AND USAGE and section WARNINGS).

ADVERSE REACTIONS

Endocrine and Urogenital, Female—The most common side effects of andro-gen therapy are amenorrhea and other menstrual irregularities, inhibition of gonadotropin secretion, and virilization, including deepening of the voice and clitoral enlargement. The latter is usually not reversible after androgens are discontinued. When administered in a pregnant woman, androgens cause vir-ilization of the external genitalia of the female fetus. Male—Gynecomastia, and excessive frequency and duration of penile erections. Oligospermia may occur at high dosages (see section CLINICAL PHARMACOLOGY).

Skin and Appendages – Hirsutism, male pattern baldness, and acne.

Fluid and Electrolyte Disturbances – Retention of sodium, chloride, water, potassium, calcium (see section WARNINGS), and inorganic phosphates.

Gastrointestinal – Nausea, cholestatic jaundice, alterations in liver function tests; rarely, hepatocellular neoplasms, peliosis hepatis (see section WARNINGS).

Hematologic – Suppression of clotting factors II, V, VII, and X; bleeding in patients on concomitant anticoagulant therapy; polycythemia.

Nervous System - Increased or decreased libido, headache, anxiety, depression, and generalized paresthesia.

Metabolic - Increased serum cholesterol.

Miscellaneous - Rarely, anaphylactoid reactions; inflammation and pain at injection site.

DRUG ABUSE AND DEPENDENCE

DELATESTRYL® (Testosterone Enanthate Injection, USP) is classified as a controlled substance under the Anabolic Steroids Control Act of 1990 and has been assigned to Schedule III.

OVERDOSAGE

There have been no reports of acute overdosage with androgens.

DOSAGE AND ADMINISTRATION

Dosage and duration of therapy with DELATESTRYL® (Testosterone Enanthate Injection, USP) will depend on age, sex, diagnosis, patient's response to treatment, and appearance of adverse effects. When properly given, injections of DELATESTRYL are well tolerated. Care should be taken to slowly inject the preparation deeply into the gluteal muscle, being sure to follow the usual precautions for intramuscular administration, such as the avoidance of intravascular injection (see section PRECAUTIONS).

In general, total doses above 400 mg/month are not required because of the prolonged action of the preparation. Injections more frequently than every 2 weeks are rarely indicated. NOTE: Use of a wet needle or a wet syringe may cause the solution to become cloudy; however, this does not affect the potency of the material. Parenteral drug products should be inspected visually for particulate matter and discoloration before administration, whenever solution and container permit. DELATESTRYL is a clear, colorless to pale yellow solution.

Male hypogonadism: As replacement therapy, i.e., for eunuchism, the suggested dosage is in the range of 50–400 mg every 2 to 4 weeks.

In males with delayed puberty: Various dosage regimens have been used; some call for lower dosages initially with gradual increases as puberty progresses, with or without a decrease to maintenance levels. Other regimens call for higher dosage to induce pubertal changes and lower dosage for maintenance after puberty. The chronological and skeletal ages must be taken into consideration, both in determining the initial dose and in adjusting the dose. Dosage is within the range of 50–200 mg every 2 to 4 weeks for a limited duration, for example, 4 to 6 months. X-rays should be taken at appropriate intervals to determine the amount of bone maturation and skeletal development (see section 6, INDICATIONS AND USAGE and section WARNINGS).

Palliation of inoperable mammary cancer in women: A dosage of 200–400 mg every 2 to 4 weeks is recommended. Women with metastatic breast carcinoma must be observed closely because androgen therapy occasionally appears to accelerate the disease.

HOW SUPPLIED

DELATESTRYL® (Testosterone Enanthate Injection, USP) is available in 5 mL (200 mg/mL) multiple dose vials.

STORAGE

DELATESTRYL® (Testosterone Enanthate Injection, USP) should be stored at room temperature. Warming and rotating the vial between the palms of the hands will re-dissolve any crystals that may have formed during storage at low temperatures.

For Prescription Use Only

PACKAGE INSERT INFORMATION FOR ANDROGEL :

FULL PRESCRIBING INFORMATION

Indications and Usage for AndroGel

1.1 Testosterone Replacement Therapy

AndroGel, an androgen, is indicated for replacement therapy in adult males for conditions associated with a deficiency or absence of endogenous testosterone:

- Primary Hypogonadism (Congenital or Acquired) - testicular failure due to cryptorchidism, bilateral torsion, orchitis, vanishing testis syndrome, orchiectomy, Klinefelter's syndrome, chemotherapy, or toxic damage from alcohol or heavy metals. These men usually have low serum testosterone levels and gonadotropins (FSH, LH) above the normal range.
- Hypogonadotropic Hypogonadism (Congenital or Acquired) - idiopathic gonadotropin or luteinizing hormone-releasing hormone (LHRH) deficiency or pituitary-hypothalamic injury from tumors, trauma, or radiation. These men have low testosterone serum levels but have gonadotropins in the normal or low range.

AndroGel Dosage and Administratio

2.1 General Dosing

The recommended starting dose of AndroGel is 5 g once daily (preferably in the morning) to clean, dry, intact skin of the shoulders and upper arms and/or abdomen. AndroGel must not be applied to the genitals. AndroGel is supplied as either a pump or in individual packets. After applying the gel, the application site should be allowed to dry for a few minutes prior to dressing. Avoid fire, flames or smoking until the gel has dried since alcohol based products, including AndroGel, are flammable. Hands should be washed with soap and water after AndroGel has been applied. [see Warnings and Precautions (5.2, 5.10)].

2.2 Administration

Multi-Dose Pump

Patients should be instructed to prime the pump before using it for the first time by fully depressing the pump mechanism (actuation) 3 times and discard this portion of the product to assure precise dose delivery. After the priming procedure, patients should completely depress the pump one time (actuation) for every 1.25 g (AndroGel Pump) of product required to achieve the daily prescribed dosage. The product may be delivered directly into the palm of the hand and then applied to the desired application sites, either one pump actuation at a time or upon completion of all pump actuations required for the daily dose. Alternatively, the product can be applied directly to the application sites. Application directly to the sites may prevent loss of product that may occur during transfer from the palm of the hand onto the application sites. Table 1 has specific dosing guidelines for adult males when the 75 g AndroGel Pump is used.

Table 1: Specific Dosing Guidelines for Using the Adult Multi-Dose Pump

Prescribed Daily Dose	Number of Pump Actuations in 75 g Pump
5 g	4 (once daily)
7.5 g	6 (once daily)
10 g	8 (once daily)

Packets

The entire contents should be squeezed into the palm of the hand and immediately applied to the application sites. Alternately, patients may squeeze a portion of the gel from the packet into the palm of the hand and apply to application sites. Repeat until entire contents have been applied.

2.3 Dose Adjustment and Patient Assessments

- To ensure proper dosing, serum testosterone levels should be measured at intervals and replaced to serum testosterone levels in the normal range. If the serum testosterone concentration is below the normal range, the daily AndroGel dose may be increased from 5 g to 7.5 g and from 7.5 g to 10 g for adult males as instructed by the physician. If the serum testosterone concentration exceeds the normal range, the daily AndroGel dose may be decreased. If the serum testosterone concentration consistently exceeds the normal range at a daily dose of 5 g, AndroGel therapy should be discontinued.

The following is general advice for treating and monitoring adult patients on AndroGel. No specific recommendations can be made.

- Prescribers should be aware that testosterone is contraindicated in men with known or suspected prostate cancer. Therefore, evaluation for prostate cancer prior to initiation of AndroGel therapy is appropriate [see Contraindications (4)].
- Based on results from controlled studies, serum PSA may rise when taking AndroGel. Therefore, periodic assessment of serum PSA is recommended in patients taking AndroGel [see Adverse Reactions (6.1)].
- Based on results from controlled studies, worsening of BPH may occur in patients taking AndroGel [see Adverse Reactions (6.1)]. Therefore, periodic assessments for signs and symptoms of BPH are recommended in patients taking AndroGel.
- Hematocrit, serum lipid profile, and liver function test should be monitored in patients taking AndroGel [see Warnings and Precautions (5.9)].

Dosage Forms and Strengths

AndroGel (testosterone gel) 1% for topical use is available in either unit-dose packets or multiple-dose pumps. The 75 g (60 metered-dose) pump delivers 1.25 g of product when the pump mechanism is fully depressed once.

AndroGel is available in the following three package containers:

- 2 x 75 g pumps (each pump dispenses 60 metered 1.25 g doses)
- 2.5 g packet
- 5 g packet

Contraindications

AndroGel should not be used in any of the following patients:

- Men with carcinoma of the breast or known or suspected carcinoma of the prostate [see Warnings and Precautions (5.1), Adverse Reactions (6.1), and Nonclinical Toxicology (13.1)].
- Women who are or may become pregnant, or who are breastfeeding. AndroGel can cause fetal harm when administered to a pregnant woman. AndroGel may cause serious adverse reactions in nursing infants. Exposure of a female fetus or nursing infant to androgens may result in varying degrees of virilization. Pregnant women or those who may become pregnant need to be aware of the potential for transfer of testosterone from men treated with AndroGel [see Warnings and Precautions (5.2) and Use in Specific Populations (8.1, 8.3)].
- Men with known hypersensitivity to any of its ingredients, including alcohol and soy products.

Warnings and Precautions

5.1 Worsening of BPH and Potential Risk of Prostate Cancer

- Patients with BPH treated with androgens are at an increased risk for worsening of signs and symptoms of BPH.
- Patients treated with androgens may be at increased risk for prostate cancer. Evaluation of the patient for prostate cancer prior to initiating and during treatment with androgens is appropriate [see Warnings and Precaution (5.9), Adverse Reactions (6.1), and Nonclinical Toxicology (13.1)].
- Increases in serum PSA from baseline values were seen in approximately 18% of individuals in an open label study of 162 hypogonadal men treated with AndroGel for up to 42 months. Most of these increases were seen within the first year of therapy [see Contraindications (4), Warnings and Precautions (5.9), Adverse Reactions (6), and Nonclinical Toxicology (13.1)].

5.2 Potential for Testosterone Transfer to Others

Transfer of testosterone to others (including women and children) can occur when vigorous skin-to-skin contact is made with the application site [see Clinical Studies (14.3)]. The following precautions are recommended to minimize potential transfer of testosterone from AndroGel-treated skin to another person:

- Patients should wash their hands immediately with soap and water after application of AndroGel.
- Patients should cover the application site(s) with clothing after the gel has dried (e.g., a shirt).
- In the event that unwashed or unclothed skin to which AndroGel has been applied does come in direct contact with the skin of another person, the general area of contact on the other person should be washed with soap and water as soon as possible. In vitro studies show that residual testosterone is removed from the skin surface by washing with soap and water.
- Women and children should avoid skin contact with AndroGel application sites in males. Changes in body hair distribution, significant increase in acne, or other signs of virilization should be brought to the attention of a physician. AndroGel may cause fetal harm in a pregnant woman due to virilization of a female fetus [see Use in Specific Populations (8.1)].

5.3 Use in Women
Due to lack of controlled evaluations in women and potential virilizing effects, AndroGel is not indicated for use in women [see Use in Specific Populations (8.1, 8.3)].

5.4 Potential for Adverse Effects on Spermatogenesis
At large doses of exogenous androgens, spermatogenesis may be suppressed through feedback inhibition of pituitary follicle-stimulating hormone (FSH) which could possibly lead to adverse effects on semen parameters including sperm count.

5.5 Hepatic Adverse Effects
Prolonged use of high doses of orally active 17-alpha-alkyl androgens (e.g., methyltestosterone) has been associated with serious hepatic adverse effects (peliosis hepatis, hepatic neoplasms, cholestatic hepatitis, and jaundice). Peliosis hepatis can be a life-threatening or fatal complication. Long-term therapy with intramuscular testosterone enanthate has produced multiple hepatic adenomas. AndroGel is not known to produce these adverse effects.

There are rare reports of hepatocellular carcinoma in patients receiving long-term oral therapy with androgens in high doses. Withdrawal of the drugs did not lead to regression of the tumors in all cases.

5.6 Edema
Drugs in the androgen class may promote retention of sodium and water. Edema with or without congestive heart failure may be a serious complication in patients with preexisting cardiac, renal, or hepatic disease [see Adverse Reactions (6.2)].

5.7 Gynecomastia
Gynecomastia may develop and may persist in patients being treated with androgens, including AndroGel, for hypogonadism.

5.8 Sleep Apnea
The treatment of hypogonadal men with testosterone products may potentiate sleep apnea in some patients, especially those with risk factors such as obesity or chronic lung diseases [see Adverse Reactions (6.2)].

5.9 Laboratory Tests

- Increases in hematocrit, reflective of increases in red blood cell mass, may require lowering or discontinuation of testosterone. Increase in red blood cell mass may increase the risk for a thromboembolic event.
- Changes in serum lipid profile may require dose adjustment or discontinuation of testosterone therapy.
- Androgens may decrease levels of thyroxin-binding globulin, resulting in decreased total T4 serum levels and increased resin uptake of T3 and T4. Free thyroid hormone levels remain unchanged, however, and there is no clinical evidence of thyroid dysfunction.
- Androgens should be used with caution in cancer patients at risk of hypercalcemia (and associated hypercalciuria). Regular monitoring of serum calcium concentrations is recommended in these patients.

5.10 Flammable until Dry

- Alcohol Based Products including AndroGel are flammable; therefore avoid fire, flame or smoking until the gel has dried.

Adverse Reactions

6.1 Clinical Trial Experience

Because clinical trials are conducted under widely varying conditions, adverse reaction rates observed in the clinical trials of a drug cannot be directly compared to rates in the clinical trials of another drug and may not reflect the rates observed in practice.

Clinical Trials in Hypogonadal Men

Table 2 shows the incidence of all adverse events judged by the investigator to be at least possibly related to treatment with AndroGel and reported by >1% of patients in a 180 Day, Phase 3 study.

Table 2: Adverse Events Possibly, Probably or Definitely Related to Use of AndroGel in the 180-Day Controlled Clinical Trial

Adverse Event	Dose of Androgel		
	5 grams N = 77	7.5 grams N = 40	10 grams N = 78
Acne	1%	3%	8%
Alopecia	1%	0%	1%
Application Site Reaction	5%	3%	4%
Asthenia	0%	3%	1%
Depression	1%	0%	1%
Emotional Lability	0%	3%	3%
Gynecomastia	1%	0%	3%
Headache	4%	3%	0%
Hypertension	3%	0%	3%
Lab Test Abnormal *	6%	5%	3%
Libido Decreased	0%	3%	1%
Nervousness	0%	3%	1%
Pain Breast	1%	3%	1%
Prostate Disorder **	3%	3%	5%
Testis Disorder ***	3%	0%	0%

* Lab test abnormal occurred in nine patients with one or more of the following events reported: elevated hemoglobin or hematocrit, hyperlipidemia, elevated triglycerides, hypokalemia, decreased HDL, elevated glucose, elevated creatinine, elevated total bilirubin.

** Prostate disorders included five patients with enlarged prostate, one with BPH, and one with elevated PSA results.

*** Testis disorders were reported in two patients: one with left varicocele and one with slight sensitivity of left testis.

Other less common adverse reactions, reported in fewer than 1% of patients included: amnesia, anxiety, discolored hair, dizziness, dry skin, hirsutism, hostility, impaired urination, paresthesia, penis disorder, peripheral edema, sweating, and vasodilation.

In this 180 day clinical trial, skin reactions at the site of application were reported with AndroGel, but none was severe enough to require treatment or discontinuation of drug.

Six patients (4%) in this trial had adverse events that led to discontinuation of AndroGel. These events included: cerebral hemorrhage, convulsion (neither of which were considered related to AndroGel administration), depression, sadness, memory loss, elevated prostate specific antigen, and hypertension No AndroGel patient discontinued due to skin reactions.

In a separate uncontrolled pharmacokinetic study of 10 patients, two had adverse events associated with AndroGel; these were asthenia and depression in one patient and increased libido and hyperkinesia in the other.

In a 3 year, flexible dose, extension study, the incidence of all adverse events judged by the investigator to be at least possibly related to treatment with AndroGel and reported by greater than 1% of patients is shown in Table 3.

Two patients reported serious adverse events considered possibly related to treatment: deep vein thrombosis (DVT) and prostate disorder requiring a transurethral resection of the prostate (TURP).

Discontinuation for adverse events in this study included: two patients with application site reactions, one with kidney failure, and five with prostate disorders (including increase in serum PSA in 4 patients, and increase in PSA with prostate enlargement in a fifth patient).

Increases in Serum PSA Observed in Clinical Trials of Hypogonadal Men

During the initial 6-month study, the mean change in PSA values had a statistically significant increase of 0.26 ng/mL. Serum PSA was measured every 6 months thereafter in the 162 hypogonadal men on AndroGel in the 3-year extension study. There was no additional statistically significant increase observed in mean PSA from 6 months through 36 months. However, there were increases in serum PSA observed in approximately 18% of individual patients. The overall mean change from baseline in serum PSA values for the entire group from month 6 to 36 was 0.11 ng/mL.

Table 3: Adverse Events Possibly, Probably or Definitely Related to Use of AndroGel in the 3 Year, Flexible Dose, Extension Study

Adverse Event	Percent of Subjects (N = 162)
Lab Test Abnormal+	9.3
Skin dry	1.9
Application Site Reaction	5.6
Acne	3.1
Pruritus	1.9
Enlarged Prostate	11.7
Carcinoma of Prostate	1.2
Urinary Symptoms*	3.7
Testis Disorder**	1.9
Gynecomastia	2.5
Anemia	2.5

+ Lab test abnormal occurred in 15 patients with one or more of the following events reported: elevated AST, elevated ALT, elevated testosterone, elevated hemoglobin or hematocrit, elevated cholesterol, elevated cholesterol/LDL ratio, elevated triglycerides, elevated HDL, elevated serum creatinine.
* Urinary symptoms included nocturia, urinary hesitancy, urinary incontinence, urinary retention, urinary urgency and weak urinary stream.
** Testis disorders included three patients. There were two with a non-palpable testis and one with slight right testicular tenderness.

Twenty-nine patients (18%) met the per-protocol criterion for increase in serum PSA, defined as greater than 2X the baseline or any single serum PSA greater than 6 ng/mL. Most of these (25/29) met this criterion by at least doubling of their PSA from baseline. In most cases where PSA at least doubled (22/25), the maximum serum PSA value was still less than 2 ng/mL. The first occurrence of a pre-specified, post-baseline increase in serum PSA was seen at or prior to Month 12 in most of the patients who met this criterion (23 of 29; 79%).

Four patients met this criterion by having a serum PSA greater than 6 ng/mL and in these, maximum serum PSA values were 6.2 ng/mL, 6.6 ng/mL, 6.7 ng/mL, and 10.7 ng/mL. In two of these patients, prostate cancer was detected on biopsy. The first patient's PSA levels were 4.7 ng/mL and 6.2 ng/mL at baseline and at Month 6/Final, respectively. The second patient's PSA levels were 4.2 ng/mL, 5.2 ng/mL, 5.8 ng/mL, and 6.6 ng/mL at baseline, Month 6, Month 12, and Final, respectively.

6.2 Postmarketing Experience

The following adverse reactions have been identified during post approval use of AndroGel. Because the reactions are reported voluntarily from a population of uncertain size, it is not always possible to reliably estimate their frequency or establish a causal relationship to drug exposure.

Hypogonadal Men

Table 4 includes adverse reactions that have been identified postmarketing.

Table 4: Adverse Drug Reactions from Postmarketing Experience of AndroGel by MedDRA System Organ Class

Blood and the lymphatic system disorders:	Elevated Hgb, Hct (polycythemia)
Endocrine disorders:	Hirsutism
Gastrointestinal disorders:	Nausea
General disorders and administration site reactions:	Asthenia, edema, malaise
Genitourinary disorders:	Impaired urination
Hepatobiliary disorders:	Abnormal liver function tests (e.g. transaminases, elevated GCTP, bilirubin)
Investigations:	Elevated PSA, electrolyte changes (nitrogen, calcium, potassium, phosphorus, sodium), changes in serum lipids (hyperlipidemia, elevated triglycerides, decreased HDL), impaired glucose tolerance, fluctuating testosterone levels, weight increase
Neoplasms benign, malignant and unspecified (cysts and polyps):	Prostate cancer
Nervous system:	Headache, dizziness, sleep apnea, insomnia
Psychiatric disorders:	Depression, emotional lability, decreased libido, nervousness, hostility, amnesia, anxiety
Reproductive system and breast disorders:	Gynecomastia, mastodynia, prostatic enlargement, testicular atrophy, oligospermia, priapism (frequent or prolonged erections)
Respiratory disorders:	Dyspnea
Skin and subcutaneous tissue disorders:	Acne, alopecia, application site reaction (pruritus, dry skin, erythema, rash, discolored hair, paresthesia), sweating
Vascular disorders:	Hypertension, vasodilation (hot flushes)

Drug Interactions

7.1 Insulin
Changes in insulin sensitivity or glycemic control may occur in patients treated with androgens. In diabetic patients, the metabolic effects of androgens may decrease blood glucose and, therefore, insulin requirements.

7.2 Corticosteroids
The concurrent use of testosterone with ACTH or corticosteroids may result in increased fluid retention and should be monitored cautiously, particularly in patients with cardiac, renal or hepatic disease.

7.3 Oral Anticoagulants
Changes in anticoagulant activity may be seen with androgens. More frequent monitoring of INR and prothrombin time are recommended in patients taking anticoagulants, especially at the initiation and termination of androgen therapy.

USE IN SPECIFIC POPULATIONS

8.1 Pregnancy
Pregnancy Category X: AndroGel is contraindicated during pregnancy or in women who may become pregnant. It is teratogenic and may cause fetal harm [see Contraindications (4)]. Exposure of a female fetus to androgens may result in varying degrees of virilization. If this drug is used during pregnancy, or if the patient becomes pregnant while taking this drug, the patient should be apprised of the potential hazard to a fetus.

8.3 Nursing Mothers
Although it is not known how much testosterone transfers into human milk, AndroGel is contraindicated in nursing women because of the potential for serious adverse reactions in nursing infants [see Contraindications (4)].
    Testosterone and other androgens may adversely affect lactation.

8.4 Pediatric Use
Safety and efficacy of AndroGel in males less than 18 years old has not been established. Improper use may result in acceleration of bone age and premature closure of epiphyses.

8.5 Geriatric Use
There have not been sufficient numbers of geriatric patients involved in controlled clinical studies utilizing AndroGel to determine whether efficacy in those over 65 years of age differs from younger subjects. Additionally, there is insufficient long-term safety data in geriatric patients to assess the potential risks of cardiovascular disease and prostate cancer.

8.6 Renal or Hepatic Impairment
No formal studies were conducted involving patients with renal or hepatic insufficiencies.

Drug Abuse and Dependence

9.1 Controlled Substance
AndroGel contains testosterone, a Schedule III controlled substance as defined by the Anabolic Steroids Control Act.

Oral ingestion of AndroGel will not result in clinically significant serum testosterone concentrations due to extensive first-pass metabolism.

Overdosage

There is one report of acute overdosage with use of an approved injectable testosterone product: this subject had serum testosterone levels of up to 11,400 ng/dL with a cerebrovascular accident. Treatment of overdosage would consist of discontinuation of AndroGel together with appropriate symptomatic and supportive care.

AndroGel Description

AndroGel (testosterone gel) 1% is a clear, colorless hydroalcoholic gel containing 1% testosterone. Topical administration of AndroGel 5 g, 7.5 g, or 10 g contains 50 mg, 75 mg, or 100 mg of testosterone, respectively, is to be applied daily to the skin's surface. Approximately 10% of the applied testosterone dose is absorbed across skin of average permeability during a 24-hour period.

The active pharmacologic ingredient in AndroGel is testosterone. Testosterone USP is a white to practically white crystalline powder chemically described as 17-beta hydroxyandrost-4-en-3-one. The structural formula is:

Testosterone

$C_{19}H_{28}O_2$ MW 288.42

Inactive ingredients in AndroGel are carbomer 980, ethanol 67.0%, isopropyl myristate, purified water, and sodium hydroxide. These ingredients are not pharmacologically active.

AndroGel - Clinical Pharmacology

12.1 Mechanism of Action

Endogenous androgens, including testosterone and dihydrotestosterone (DHT), are responsible for the normal growth and development of the male sex organs and for maintenance of secondary sex characteristics. These effects include the growth and maturation of prostate, seminal vesicles, penis and scrotum; the development of male hair distribution, such as facial, pubic, chest and axillary hair; laryngeal enlargement, vocal chord thickening, alterations in body musculature and fat distribution. Testosterone and DHT are necessary for the normal development of secondary sex characteristics. Male hypogonadism results from insufficient secretion of testosterone and is characterized by low serum testosterone concentrations. Signs/symptoms associated with male hypogonadism include erectile dysfunction and decreased sexual desire, fatigue and loss of energy, mood depression, regression of secondary sexual characteristics and osteoporosis.

Male hypogonadism has two main etiologies. Primary hypogonadism is caused by defects of the gonads, such as Klinefelter's Syndrome or Leydig cell aplasia, whereas secondary hypogonadism is the failure of the hypothalamus (or pituitary) to produce sufficient gonadotropins (FSH, LH).

12.3 Pharmacokinetics

Adult Males

Absorption
AndroGel delivers physiologic amounts of testosterone, producing circulating testosterone concentrations that approximate normal levels (298 – 1043 ng/dL) seen in healthy men. AndroGel provides continuous transdermal delivery of testosterone for 24 hours following a single application to intact, clean, dry skin of the shoulders, upper arms and/or abdomen.

AndroGel is a hydroalcoholic formulation that dries quickly when applied to the skin surface. The skin serves as a reservoir for the sustained release of testosterone into the systemic circulation. Approximately 10% of the testosterone dose applied on the skin surface from AndroGel is absorbed into systemic circulation. Therefore, 5 g and 10 g of AndroGel systemically deliver approximately 5 mg and 10 mg of testosterone, respectively. In a study with 10 g of AndroGel, all patients showed an increase in serum testosterone within 30 minutes, and eight of nine patients had a serum testosterone concentration within normal range by 4 hours after the initial application. Absorption of testosterone into the blood continues for the entire 24-hour dosing interval. Serum concentrations approximate the steady-state level by the end of the first 24 hours and are at steady state by the second or third day of dosing.

Figure 1: Mean (± SD) Steady-State Serum Testosterone Concentrations on Day 30 in Patients Applying AndroGel Once Daily

With single daily applications of AndroGel, follow-up measurements 30, 90 and 180 days after starting treatment have confirmed that serum testosterone concentrations are generally maintained within the eugonadal range. Figure 1summarizes the 24-hour pharmacokinetic profiles of testosterone for hypogonadal men (less than 300 ng/dL) maintained on 5 g or 10 g of AndroGel for 30 days. The average (± SD) daily testosterone concentration produced by AndroGel 10 g on Day 30 was 792 (± 294) ng/dL and by AndroGel 5 g 566 (± 262) ng/dL.

When AndroGel treatment is discontinued after achieving steady state, serum testosterone levels remain in the normal range for 24 to 48 hours but return to their pretreatment levels by the fifth day after the last application.

Distribution

Circulating testosterone is primarily bound in the serum to sex hormone-binding globulin (SHBG) and albumin. Approximately 40% of testosterone in plasma is bound to SHBG, 2% remains unbound (free) and the rest is bound to albumin and other proteins.

Metabolism

There is considerable variation in the half-life of testosterone as reported in the literature, ranging from 10 to 100 minutes. Testosterone is metabolized to various 17-keto steroids through two different pathways. The major active metabolites of testosterone are estradiol and DHT.

DHT concentrations increased in parallel with testosterone concentrations during AndroGel treatment. After 180 days of treatment in adult males, mean DHT concentrations were within the normal range with 5 g AndroGel and were about 7% above the normal range after a 10 g dose. The mean steady-state DHT/T ratio during 180 days of AndroGel treatment remained within normal limits and ranged from 0.23 to 0.29 (5 g/day) and from 0.27 to 0.33 (10 g/day).

Excretion

About 90% of a dose of testosterone given intramuscularly is excreted in the urine as glucuronic and sulfuric acid conjugates of testosterone and its metabolites; about 6% of a dose is excreted in the feces, mostly in the unconjugated form. Inactivation of testosterone occurs primarily in the liver.

NONCLLINICAL TOXICOLOGY

13.1 Carcinogenesis, Mutagenesis, Impairment of Fertility
Testosterone has been tested by subcutaneous injection and implantation in mice and rats. In mice, the implant induced cervical-uterine tumors, which metastasized in some cases. There is suggestive evidence that injection of testosterone into some strains of female mice increases their susceptibility to hepatoma. Testosterone is also known to increase the number of tumors and decrease the degree of differentiation of chemically induced carcinomas of the liver in rats.

Clinical Studies

14.1 Clinical Trials in Adult Hypogonadal Males
AndroGel was evaluated in a multi-center, randomized, parallel-group, active-controlled, 180-day trial in 227 hypogonadal men. The study was conducted in 2 phases. During the Initial Treatment Period (Days 1-90), 73 patients were randomized to AndroGel 5 g daily, 78 patients to AndroGel 10 g daily, and 76 patients to a non-scrotal testosterone transdermal system. The study was double-blind for dose of AndroGel but open-label for active control. Patients who were originally randomized to AndroGel and who had single-sample serum testosterone levels above or below the normal range on Day 60 were titrated to 7.5 g daily on Day 91. During the Extended Treatment Period (Days 91-180), 51 patients continued on AndroGel 5 g daily, 52 patients continued on AndroGel 10 g daily, 41 patients continued on a non-scrotal testosterone transdermal system (5 mg daily), and 40 patients received AndroGel 7.5 g daily. Upon completion of the initial study, 163 enrolled and 162 patients received treatment in an open-label extension study of AndroGel for an additional period of up to 3 years.

Mean peak, trough and average serum testosterone concentrations within the normal range (298-1043 ng/dL) were achieved on the first day of treatment with doses of 5 g and 10 g. In patients continuing on AndroGel 5 g and 10 g, these mean testosterone levels were maintained within the normal range for the 180-day duration of the original study. Figure 2 summarizes the 24-hour pharmacokinetic profiles of testosterone administered as AndroGel for 30, 90 and 180 days. Testosterone concentrations were maintained as long as the patient continued to properly apply the prescribed AndroGel treatment.

Figure 2: Mean Steady-State Testosterone Concentrations in Patients with Once-Daily AndroGel Therapy

Table 5 summarizes the mean testosterone concentrations on Treatment Day 180 for patients receiving 5 g, 7.5 g, or 10 g of AndroGel. The 7.5 g dose produced mean concentrations intermediate to those produced by 5 g and 10 g of AndroGe.

Table 5: Mean (± SD) Steady-State Serum Testosterone Concentrations During Therapy (Day 180)

	5 g	7.5 g	10 g
	N = 44	N = 37	N = 48
Cavg	555 ± 225	601 ± 309	713 ± 209
Cmax	830 ± 347	901 ± 471	1083 ± 434
Cmin	371 ± 165	406 ± 220	485 ± 156

Of 129 hypogonadal men who were appropriately titrated with AndroGel and who had sufficient data for analysis, 87% achieved an average serum testosterone level within the normal range on Treatment Day 180.

In patients treated with AndroGel, there were no observed differences in the average daily serum testosterone concentrations at steady-state based on age, cause of hypogonadism, or body mass index.

AndroGel 5 g/day and 10 g/day resulted in significant increases over time in total body mass and total body lean mass, while total body fat mass and the percent body fat decreased significantly. These changes were maintained for 180 days of treatment during the original study. Changes in the 7.5 g dose group were similar. Bone mineral density in both hip and spine increased significantly from Baseline to Day 180 with 10 g AndroGel.

AndroGel treatment at 5 g/day and 10 g/day for 90 days produced significant improvement in libido (measured by sexual motivation, sexual activity and enjoyment of sexual activity as assessed by patient responses to a questionnaire). The degree of penile erection as subjectively estimated by the patients, increased with AndroGel treatment, as did the subjective score for "satisfactory duration of erection." AndroGel treatment at 5 g/day and 10 g/day produced positive effects on mood and fatigue. Similar changes were seen after 180 days of treatment and in the group treated with the 7.5 g dose. DHT concentrations increased in parallel with testosterone concentrations at AndroGel doses of 5 g/day and 10 g/day, but the DHT/T ratio stayed within the normal range, indicating enhanced availability of the major physiologically active androgen. Serum estradiol (E2) concentrations increased significantly within 30 days of starting treatment with AndroGel 5 or 10 g/day and remained elevated throughout the treatment period but remained within the normal range for eugonadal men. Serum levels of SHBG decreased very slightly (1 to 11%) during AndroGel treatment. In men with hypergonadotropic hypogonadism, serum levels of LH and FSH fell in a dose- and time-dependent manner during treatment with AndroGel.

14.2 Phototoxicity in Humans

The phototoxic potential of AndroGel was evaluated in a double-blind, single-dose study in 27 subjects with photosensitive skin types. The Minimal Erythema Dose (MED) of ultraviolet radiation was determined for each subject. A single 24 (+1) hour application of duplicate patches containing test articles (placebo gel, testosterone gel, or saline) was made to naive skin sites on Day 1. On Day 2, each subject received five exposure times of ultraviolet radiation, each exposure being 25% greater than the previous one. Skin evaluations were made on Days 2 to 5. Exposure of test and control article application sites to ultraviolet light did not produce increased inflammation relative to non-irradiated sites, indicating no phototoxic effect.

14.3 Testosterone Transfer from Male Patients to Female Partners
The potential for dermal testosterone transfer following AndroGel use was evaluated in a clinical study between males dosed with AndroGel and their untreated female partners. Two (2) to 12 hours after AndroGel (10 g) application by the male subjects, the couples (N = 38 couples) engaged in daily, 15-minute sessions of vigorous skin-to-skin contact so that the female partners gained maximum exposure to the AndroGel application sites. Under these study conditions, all unprotected female partners had a serum testosterone concentration greater than 2 times the baseline value at some time during the study. When a shirt covered the application site(s), the transfer of testosterone from the males to the female partners was completely prevented.

How Supplied/Storage and Handling
AndroGel is supplied in non-aerosol, metered-dose pumps. The pump is composed of plastic and stainless steel and an LDPE/aluminum foil inner liner encased in rigid plastic with a polypropylene cap. Each 88 g AndroGel Pump in the twin package is capable of dispensing 75 g or 60 metered 1.25 g doses.

AndroGel is also supplied in unit-dose aluminum foil packets in cartons of 30. Each packet of 2.5 g or 5 g gel contains 25 mg or 50 mg testosterone, respectively.

NDC Number	Package Size
54868-5814-0	2 x 75 g pumps (each pump dispenses 60 metered 1.25 g doses)
54868-4792-0	30 packets (2.5 g per packet)
54868-4810-0	30 packets (5 g per packet)

Keep AndroGel out of the reach of children.

Storage

Store at 25°C (77°F); excursions permitted to 15° to 30°C (59° to 86°F) [see USP Controlled Room Temperature].

Disposal
Used AndroGel pumps or used AndroGel packets should be discarded in
household trash in a manner that prevents accidental application or ingestion by children or pets.

Patient Counseling Information
See FDA-approved patient labeling (17.3)

17.1 Potential Adverse Reactions with Androgens
Patients should be informed that treatment with androgens may lead to
adverse reactions which include:

- Changes in urinary habits such as increased urination at night, trouble
  starting your urine stream, passing urine many times during the day,
  having an urge that you have to go to the bathroom right away, having
  a urine accident, being unable to pass urine and weak urine flow.
- Breathing disturbances, including those associated with sleep, or excessive daytime sleepiness.
- Too frequent or persistent erections of the penis.
- Nausea, vomiting, changes in skin color, or ankle swelling.

17.2 Instructions for Use of AndroGel

- Patients should be informed to apply AndroGel once daily (preferably
  in the morning) to clean, dry skin of the shoulders and upper arms and/
  or abdomen. To prevent transfer of AndroGel to others, patient should
  wash their hands after application and cover the application site with
  clothing.
- Advise patients that AndroGel is an alcohol based product and is flammable, therefore avoid fire, flame or smoking until the gel has dried.
- Counsel patients on the importance of adhering to all recommended
  monitoring by their healthcare professional.
- Advise patients to report any changes in their state of health, such as
  changes in urinary habits, breathing, sleep, and mood.

17.3 FDA-Approved Patient Labeling
AndroGel (testosterone gel) 1% CIII is available packaged with 2 x 75 g
pumps (each pump dispenses 60 metered 1.25 g doses) or in a box of 30
packets with 2.5g or 5g gel.

This is a summary of the important information about AndroGel. For details, talk to your healthcare professional and refer to the package insert.

1. What Disease or Condition Does AndroGel Treat?
Your healthcare provider has prescribed this medication because your body does not produce enough testosterone. The medical term for this condition is hypogonadism.

2. How Should AndroGel (Pump or Packet) Be Applied?
It is important that you use AndroGel as prescribed by your healthcare professional. If you experience serious problems, contact your healthcare professional. Your healthcare professional will tell you how much AndroGel to use each day.

Men should apply gel to starred (upper arm/shoulders) or shaded (abdomen) areas only.

Figure3: Site(s) of Gel Application

- AndroGel should be applied once daily at the same time each day (preferably every morning) to clean, dry, healthy, intact skin of the shoulders, upper arms and/or abdomen. If you take a bath or shower in the morning, use AndroGel after your bath or shower.
- AndroGel should not be applied to the penis or scrotum, or to skin with open sores, wounds or irritation.
- Wash your hands with soap and water immediately after application to reduce the chance that the medication will spread from your hands to other people.

- Let AndroGel dry for a few minutes before you dress.
- AndroGel is flammable until dry; allow the gel to dry before smoking or going near an open flame.
- Wait 5 to 6 hours before showering or swimming. This will ensure that the greatest amount of AndroGel is absorbed into your system.

How to use the AndroGel pump?
It is important that you read and follow these directions on how to use the AndroGel Pump properly. Before using the pump for the first time, you must prime the AndroGel pump by fully depressing the pump three times and discarding the gel. The unused gel should be discarded in a manner to avoid accidental exposure or ingestion by household members or pets. Fully depress the pump the appropriate number of times to deliver the daily dose prescribed by your healthcare provider. The product may be delivered directly into the palm of your hand and then applied to the desired application sites, either one pump depression at a time or upon completion of all pump depressions required for the daily dose.

How to use the AndroGel packets?
Open one AndroGel aluminum foil packet by folding the top edge at the perforation and tearing completely across the packet along the perforation. Squeeze the contents into the palm of your hand. Squeeze from the bottom of the packet toward the top. If you like, you may squeeze a portion of the gel from the packet into the palm of your hand and apply to application site(s). Repeat until the entire contents of the packet have been applied.

3. What Should You Discuss With Your Healthcare Professional?
Before you start using AndroGel, tell your healthcare professional if you :

- Have prostate cancer or breast cancer.
- Have a known hypersensitivity to any of AndroGel's components, including individuals who are hypersensitive to testosterone that is chemically synthesized from soy.

4. What Other Drugs Should Not Be Used Together With AndroGel?
Tell your healthcare provider about all of the medicines you take, including prescription and non-prescription medicines, vitamins and herbal supplements. AndroGel can affect how your body handles other drugs. Changes in your dose or careful monitoring may be needed if you are taking any of the following medications:

- Insulin
- Corticosteroids
- Oral Anticoagulants

5. What Are the Side Effects and Risks?

Possible side effects of AndroGel to discuss with your healthcare professional include:

Most common: Skin irritation where gel is applied, breast development or tenderness, acne, prostate enlargement, changes in lab test results and changes in urinary habits.

Contact your healthcare professional if you experience any of the following adverse reactions:

- Too frequent or persistent erections of the penis.
- Any nausea, vomiting, changes in skin color or ankle swelling.
- Breathing disturbances, including those associated with sleep, or excessive daytime sleepiness.
- Changes in urinary habits such as increased urination at night, trouble starting your urine stream, passing urine many times during the day, having an urge that you have to go to the bathroom right away, having a urine accident, being unable to pass urine and weak urine flow.

The major risks of AndroGel include:

Prostate Disorders: Patients treated with testosterone may be at an increased risk for prostate enlargement, and prostate cancer. Talk to your healthcare provider for more information on risk factors and ways to monitor for prostate disorders.   Testosterone Transfer: Transfer of testosterone to others (including women and children) can occur when vigorous skin-to-skin contact is made with the application site. AndroGel must not be used by women, and exposure to the active ingredient testosterone in pregnancy can cause fetal harm. Notify your healthcare provider if your female partner develops changes in hair distribution, increases in acne or other signs of masculinity.

6. How Should AndroGel Be Stored?

Store at 25°C (77°F); excursions permitted to 15° to 30°C (59° to 86°F) [see USP Controlled Room Temperature]. Keep out of the reach of children.

7. Is there Anything Else I Need to Know When Using AndroGel?
Your healthcare professional has prescribed AndroGel to meet your specific needs; never share your AndroGel with anyone. If you have any questions or concerns about your AndroGel treatment, ask your healthcare provider or pharmacist.